STOKING THE FIRE
A Surgical Memoir of London

By

Charles Stewart Roberts, MD

Assistant Professor of Surgery
Division of Cardiothoracic Surgery
Department of Surgery
The University of North Carolina
Chapel Hill, North Carolina

FUTURA

Futura Publishing Company, Inc.
Armonk, NY

Library of Congress Cataloging-in-Publication Data

Roberts, Charles Stewart
Stoking the fire : a surgical memoir of London / by Charles Stewart Roberts.
p. cm.
Includes bibliographical references.
ISBN 0–87993–422–0
1. Roberts, Charles Stewart. 2. Lincoln, Christopher. 3. Surgeons—United States—Biography. 4. Surgeons—Great Britain—Biography. 5. London (England)—Description and travel.
I. Title
[DNLM: 1. Roberts, Charles Stewart. 2. Lincoln, Christopher. 3. Thoracic Surgery personal narratives. WZ 100R643S 1998]
RD27.34.R58 1998
617′.092′2—dc21
DNLM/DLC
for Library of Congress 98-36943
CIP

Published by
Futura Publishing Company, Inc.
135 Bedford Road
Armonk, New York 10504–0635

L.C. #98–36943
ISBN #0–87993–422–0

Printed in the United States of America on acid-free paper.

To my Bride
Lydia Warren Roberts

Acknowledgments

This experience in London would have been impossible, had not my father so generously maintained certain financial responsibilities of mine in the States. Not knowing where Great Britain was on the globe, my little daughters, Amelia and Camille, knew their father was not in Chapel Hill and would not continue to visit regularly. For their patience and understanding, I am grateful. Part of the purpose of this book was to be able to share with them in years to come my experience abroad. They will visit London one day, and I will be interested in their own observations. Judit Farkas, a surgical assistant in Chapel Hill and wife of my colleague, Dr. Frank Detterbeck, kindly gave me a beautiful leather-bound journal, in which I entered notes during the year. My thanks also go to Ms. Betsy Mann of the University of North Carolina, who kindly typed this manuscript. Several family members and friends reviewed the manuscript and encouraged me to persist until its publication. Any author knows the importance of this encouragement. The cost of publication was partially defrayed by a generous grant from the Max and Victoria Dreyfus Foundation, based in White Plains, New York.

Preface

This book is primarily about two people: Mr. Christopher Lincoln and me. Lincoln was a Consultant Cardiothoracic Surgeon at the Royal Brompton Hospital in London, and I was his Fellow, or apprentice, for a year, from August 1996 through July 1997. Lincoln was 63 years of age and had been a consultant at the Brompton for 23 years. He was a distinguished *pediatric* cardiac surgeon, in particular, and that expertise is what prompted me to apply to train under him. I knew his personality was formidable, having interacted with him briefly in London in 1994.

At 36 years of age, I had trained in surgery for a decade in American institutions, including two years in the Surgery Branch of the National Heart, Lung, and Blood Institute, in Bethesda, and three years in the Division of Cardiothoracic Surgery at the University of North Carolina at Chapel Hill, under Dr. Benson R. Wilcox. After a year with Lincoln in London, I intended to return to the States to begin a career in academic cardiothoracic surgery.

Soon after my arrival in London, Lincoln and I were conversing in his office when he described training in surgery as "stoking the fire." He moved his arms back and forth as if shoveling coal into a furnace. A surgeon must tend the fire a sufficient period of time, grow accustomed to the heat. It would be a year of cardiac surgery, standing over the heart, "stoking the fire."

This book is an account of surgical training under Lincoln, but it is also a glimpse of life in London, as I saw it, for a year near the end of the century. Before writing a book on pellagra in 1912, my grandfather, Dr. Stewart R. Roberts, spent time in Italy studying the ravages of that nutritional disease there. He also made his way to London and Edinburgh. Though he published many papers, he left no personal account of his experience abroad, which would have interested me greatly. I was determined to record my own foreign experience.

Contents

Acknowledgments iv
Preface v

1 Meeting Lincoln 1
2 Neville Street 5
3 Lincoln in Daily Life 13
4 Royal Brompton Hospital 21
5 The Surgical Trainees 29
6 The Other American 41
7 Brompton History 45
8 Lincoln at Work 49
9 Monday Morning Conference 57
10 Wednesday Grand Rounds 59
11 Park Walk 63
12 Dr. Wilcox's Visit 71
13 St. Luke's Street 75
14 Views of America 79
15 English Cuisine 85
16 The London Language 91
17 Harley Street and the Wellington 99
18 Moraes and Chauvoud 105
19 Prague, Dublin, Hamburg 111
20 Other British Surgeons 119
21 Spring Visitors 127
22 Lincoln and Kirklin 135
23 The Bristol Affair 139
24 Medicolegal Matters 143
25 Home and Back 147
26 Stoking the Fire 151
27 Former Trainees of Lincoln 155
28 The Wedding and Departure 161

Appendix I 165
Appendix II 179
Appendix III 181

Photo section following page 184.

"I mentioned that I was afraid I put into my journal too many little incidents." JOHNSON: "There is nothing, Sir, too little for so little a creature as man. It is by studying little things that we attain the great art of having as little misery and as much happiness as possible."

James Boswell
The Life of Samuel Johnson

Chapter 1

Meeting Lincoln

That Mr. Christopher Lincoln was an extraordinary teacher of surgery was first apparent to me when I assisted him at several cardiac operations in London in April 1994. At that time, I was in my first year of a three-year training program in cardiothoracic surgery at The University of North Carolina at Chapel Hill (hereafter UNC). My chief at UNC, Dr. Benson R. Wilcox, had arranged for each first-year trainee in his program to spend two or three weeks in the laboratory of Professor Robert H. Anderson at the Royal Brompton Hospital (hereafter RBH). It was the highlight of my first year, which was otherwise spent in research in lung transplantation.

A world-renowned cardiac morphologist, Professor Anderson specialized in congenital heart defects and had accumulated and stored a large number of heart specimens that one could examine. The purpose of the London visit was to educate oneself further in congenital heart disease. After two weeks of attending courses and studying many heart specimens, I was eager to visit the operating rooms of the RBH.

Anderson kindly informed Lincoln of the presence of an American surgical trainee in his laboratory, and Lincoln called one afternoon. "Mr. Roberts, this is Mr. Lincoln. Will you assist me tomorrow on an operation?" "Yes, of course," I replied. "Good, I'll see you tomorrow in theater at 8:30. Thank you." Click. He had several operations scheduled that day and was short on assistants.

When I introduced myself the next morning, Lincoln said, "You Carolinians are always so tall must be something in the air." This amused me. Before scrubbing in to assist Lincoln, I informed him that I had completed training in general surgery *only* and had minimal experience in cardiac surgery. While I had forgotten this remark, Lincoln told me three years later that he liked its candor. During the four operations in which I assisted him over the next two days, Lincoln's engaging personality shone forth much as it would three years later when I spent a year with him.

At one operation, the second assistant surgeon was from Cuba, the anesthetist was Polish, a cardiologist with an echo machine was from Germany, and the scrub nurse was from Penang, an island off the west coast of Malaysia. "This is a world event!" Lincoln exclaimed. He commented later on Penang as "the pearl of the Orient . . . beautiful women there," and also remarked on the beauty of women of the southeastern United States, which I confirmed. He thought Southerners spoke Old English, "the way English was formerly spoken." Lincoln commented favorably on his year at the Massachusetts General Hospital in 1968 and also on the renowned Dr. John W. Kirklin of Alabama, who had "a twinkle in his eye," he said. Another American surgeon he described as having "no humanism."

Lincoln instructed at nearly every step of the operation and often gave credit to his various teachers of surgery. "Senning taught me this," he would say, or "Ross showed me this technique." The perfusionist had persuaded Lincoln to change his usual technique of arresting the heart at operation. Rather than delivering cardioplegia ("CP" as he called it) into the aortic root by passive infusion with gravity, he was persuaded to deliver the solution by active infusion with a roller pump. While measuring the pressure in the aortic root during this different technique, Lincoln became agitated, and I remember he kept repeating, "Scientific surgery . . . scientific surgery." He later reverted to the gravity method.

After three weeks in London, I returned to UNC and completed my training in cardiothoracic surgery. After the laboratory year, the second year was devoted to general thoracic surgery, primarily lung and esophageal operations, and the final year was devoted exclusively to cardiac surgery, both pediatric and adult. Because I was particularly interested in pediatric cardiac surgery, Dr. Wilcox advised me to spend an extra year of training with Lincoln at the RBH, to gain further experience. While clinical training at UNC involved two years under five surgeons, training in London would be one year under one surgeon, which would be a novel experience after a decade of American surgical training.

And so in early 1995, I wrote to Lincoln, asking if a training opportunity with him was available. Lincoln accepted me as a "Fellow in Pediatric Cardiac Surgery" to begin August 1, 1996, one month after my UNC training ended. During my last year at UNC, I read three or four plays by Shakespeare and studied a little book on British kings and queens in preparation. Another book by Ralph Waldo Emerson called *English Traits* gave some insight into the English temperament, at least as it appeared to the Anglophile, Emerson, a century and a half ago.

I had visited the UK four times during my first 36 years of life, but the visits had been brief, and I had no real knowledge of how one actually lives outside the USA. Although I admired England more than any foreign country, it was unexamined admiration. Didn't everyone admire the English? When my brother and I, in our youth, were not arranging Confederate and Union toy soldiers on the field of battle, we were lining up the Americans against the Redcoats. It never struck me as unusual that I had been to England three times before I had been west of the Mississippi River. One studied English and American literature separately and exclusively. Notwithstanding this bent toward the British Isles, my American heritage and habits extended back to Virginia, nearly four centuries ago. I was not unaware of this perspective when my American Airlines plane landed in London on July 29, 1996.

Chapter 2

Neville Street

Arriving on a Monday morning, I spent the first three days settling into a flat (apartment) in a townhouse at 2 Neville Street, a block from the hospital. Owned by the RBH, it was a two-story (street level and basement level), two-bedroom flat which was sparsely furnished. Coincidentally, it was the same flat in which Dr. and Mrs. Wilcox had lived during an eight-month sabbatical from UNC in 1980. Because this hospital flat was too big and the cost far exceeded my budget, however, I quickly made an arrangement with the Accommodations Office to move to a single room at 19 Neville Street, which was a five-level townhouse shared by several other foreign physicians. The room became my home for six months.

My first act in London was to call Judy Wilson, an American living in London whom I had never met. Her husband was Cyrus Wilson, a step-brother by marriage of Tish O'Brien, a close friend of my mother in Maryland. Notwithstanding this distant connection to me, the Wilsons were hospitable and helpful beyond words. We became friends quickly, and I was a regular visitor to their lovely town home on Park Walk in Chelsea. Cyrus Wilson, a former West Point Military Academy cadet, was a businessman with an expertise in marketing, employed by Price Waterhouse, the accounting firm. Judy knew London inside and out and had great enthusiasm for life in Britain. Theirs was the only home I entered in London that offered bourbon, an American touch of hospitality.

My single room on Neville Street was on street level with a large front window and a fireplace, over the mantel of which was a large mirror. The single bed had an excessively soft mattress. A narrow desk faced out the window, and there was a dresser, a large wooden wardrobe container, and a small table. I bought a simple lamp and an iron. Judy

Wilson brought a long pot containing flowers, which I put outside in the front window mantel.

I assumed control of a cabinet of kitchen shelves by filling them with groceries. My Grecian housemate had identified her section with a postcard of a Greek island, so I taped up to my cabinet a postcard of the rolling hills of western North Carolina. My room was adjacent to the kitchen, which was the focal point of the house. Most of the doctors cooked and ate dinner there, each at different times.

Becoming acquainted with my housemates was easy, as they were all friendly. Living at the very top of the house was Dr. Kyriaki (Kiki) Zeibecoglou, a chest physician (pulmonologist) from Greece who was pursuing a Ph.D. in immunology. Her particular research interest was the eosinophil, a type of white blood cell about which she was constantly reading, sometimes in the sun in the back garden. During that summer, she dated a German surgical trainee, Dr. Christoph Stamm, from Göttingen, with whom I became friends. The daily summer Promenade concerts were ongoing at the Royal Albert Hall, and Christoph gave me a spare ticket. On that hot August evening, the Oslo orchestra played Rossini and Mahler. Applause brought them back for three encores.

Devoted to her mother and two brothers in Greece, Kiki struggled with the idea of devoting several years to medical research in London, when her real desire was to be a clinician near her family in Greece. Both of my parents met her on separate visits and were immediately impressed by her. She had a sparkle in her eyes and took an enthusiastic interest in their visit. Once I showed her a picture of my two little daughters, and from then on, she asked me about them regularly. On Saturdays, she occasionally cooked a Greek casserole in the morning and invited me to enjoy it with her at dinner. Every Tuesday night, she would sit in the kitchen and await telephone calls from Greece. One of her two brothers died of cancer in Greece during that fall, which prompted her to return home. Her other brother was a sailor at sea. In February, when we were all asked to evacuate the townhouse, Kiki moved to a flat in North London where the Greek community was situated. Regrettably, we conversed less and less as the year passed.

Stefan Anker lived in a basement bedroom. A physically large, blond, blue-eyed German from East Berlin, he was studying heart failure under Professor Andrew J.S. Coats at the RBH. Quite successful from a publications standpoint, his particular interest was cachexia, or physical wasting, which is sometimes associated with heart failure. Our conversation usually revolved around his most recent paper. "Have you heard from *The Lancet* about your manuscript?" I would ask. His energy and enthusiasm for research were admirable.

Stefan would go regularly to Berlin on weekends to see his wife and two children, bringing back fresh bread, because he "could not stand English bread." He slept late and worked late, appearing in the kitchen at about 11 p.m. to fix dinner. His little transistor radio was always set to heavy metal rock and roll, the sound of which would penetrate my room, where I was often reading. He usually made omelets into which he put ham and cheese and onions, and his appetite was enormous. He kept a complete stock of alcoholic beverages and usually got down two Heineken beers before retiring at midnight.

On more than one occasion, Stefan asserted that he was an atheist. "I do not believe in God," he would say, and then express a version of the survival of the fittest theory. I inquired about his parents' beliefs, and he responded that his parents were also atheists. His career goal was to become a professor of heart failure in Berlin, in which he will no doubt succeed. Though he was quite open and generous in his invitation to me to visit Berlin or join him for dinner in London, I saw him only rarely after moving out of the townhouse in February. We threatened each other with a chess match, a sort of a World War III, but never played.

The third housemate whom I came to know was Eugene (Gene) Liu, an anesthetist (anesthesiologist) in training from Singapore. Slim and animated, Gene occasionally dined in the kitchen with a petite and polite Oriental nurse who worked in the recovery room. I enjoyed watching him prepare dinner, usually fried chicken or fish, with rice flavored with all sorts of spices, and I enjoyed watching him eat it, which was done with relish. In January, Gene went to Nepal for six months, before returning to Singapore to begin his consultant career. Lincoln knew something about nearly all the anesthetic trainees who passed through the RBH, because he would often question them about their past and their plans. When Gene was the anesthetist above the ether screen, Lincoln would say, "Gene and I are going to Nepal together, aren't we, Gene?"

At various times during my first six months, people stayed in the spare bedrooms of the townhouse, but my acquaintance with them was brief. A young German gynecologist and his wife stayed briefly in the flat above me for several days and attended the summer Promenade concerts each night. When they spoke of music, I fell silent, as their knowledge was broad and deep. They knew the names of specific conductors in various European cities and confidently rated the quality of each performance at the Royal Albert Hall.

Stefan Anker, the East German housemate, and Christoph Stamm, the West German boyfriend of Kiki, also knew considerably more about classical music than I. The differences in East and West Germany were probably personified in some ways in these two men. Stefan was smart and generous, and yet simple in manner. He seemed less cosmopolitan than his Western countryman.

The walls of my room I covered with maps of Europe, Italy, Germany, and London. On the wall directly beside my bed, I placed a large, colorful map of Great Britain and Ireland. If I lay awake after a difficult day, my gaze would turn to the right and focus on the names of the shires and towns of England. Later, I wrote in the names of great literary figures to associate the writer with the county: D. H. Lawrence with Derby, Samuel Johnson with Stafford, A. E. Housman with Shropshire, Shakespeare with Warwick, etc. This geographic knowledge was helpful, because during the year, Lincoln would frequently turn to me at a patient's bedside and say, "Charles, did you hear that accent?" And then back to the patient: "Say that again . . . . He is from Somerset."

During the first days in London, my five senses were bombarded. I had to grow accustomed to the dense population. As the 25th largest metropolitan area in the world in 1996, London had 7.6 million people. In the States, only New York (#4) and Los Angeles (#7) exceeded it in population. The ever-present noise of the city was new to my ears. In Chapel Hill, I had lived in the home of a widow who had five acres of rose gardens surrounded by woods. The sounds of nature came through open windows at night; now it was the clamor of the London streets. I was still reading a history of General Hood's campaign in Tennessee at the close of the Civil War, and it took me back to the States each night during the first week in England. Thereafter, for the most part, I read things English.

In London, I had to relearn several basics of daily life—how to telephone someone, where to wash clothes, what the money was worth, where to eat, how to cross streets. Getting accustomed to the flow of traffic is no light matter. My father knew a physician who was badly injured crossing a street, shortly after arriving in London. For 30 years I looked to the left, then right. Now I was supposed to look to the right, then left. Lincoln told me he had a near-death experience in Paris. As he was stepping onto a street, he looked to the right as one does in London, and a large bus came down the road from the left, brushing his nose.

On day two I went to the Royal College of Surgeons downtown at Lincoln's Inn Fields, where I was interviewed by a pleasant Englishwoman named Ann Veasey, who administered the "Overseas Doctors

Training Scheme." The word "scheme" is used many times, where "program" would be used in the States. I was to be insured only for work under Lincoln. This technicality was ignored through the year, however, as I soon rotated on the call duty schedule of the RBH, covering patients of all the surgeons, and occasionally operating with other surgeons.

While at the Royal College of Surgeons building, I toured the Hunterian Museum, the first of several visits in the year. Appearing on one wall was a plaque honoring the father of American surgery, Dr. Philip Syng Physic (1768–1837), donated by Dr. George F. Sheldon, the Chairman of the Department of Surgery at UNC. He had asked me to photograph the plaque for him, and I did so. Sheldon was interested in John Hunter, particularly his influence on American surgery, about which Sheldon later wrote an extensive article.

Also on the second day, I went to the "Aliens Registration Office" in a police station on "Lamb's Conduit Street." The scene in the building was something one might imagine in Calcutta in 1910. There was a long table with at least twenty bureaucrats seated in a row facing "aliens" seated opposite in chairs. One made it to a chair only after a long wait in line on a lower level. I handed a man documents, and then he started stamping things. I learned early in the year that the British love to stamp things. They stamp everything you give them at the bank, except money. Each time I would pick up my monthly salary at the cashier's office at the RBH, a clerk would stamp two or three documents.

On my third day in London, I appeared at the RBH to let Lincoln know that I had arrived and planned to begin the next day, August 1. "You're taller than I," was his first remark, similar to his statement three years earlier. We talked for about an hour in his office, and I was introduced to Melanie Cheung, his highly talented secretary. I gave Lincoln a copy of *The Adventures of Huckleberry Finn,* the great American novel, which may collect dust on his shelf. The next day I rose at 6 a.m. and began work.

From July through September, Dr. D. Luke Glancy, my father's best friend, was also at the RBH. While chief of cardiology at Louisiana State University in New Orleans, he had decided to take a six-month sabbatical, the first three months in London and the second three months in Florida. In London, he spent most of his time with Dr. Jane Somerville, the world-renowned expert in congenital heart disease in adults. Glancy analyzed all the operations on adults with congenital heart disease at the RBH, a study that was later published in *The American Journal of Cardiology* (Dore A, Glancy DL, Stone S, Menashe VD, Somerville J: Cardiac surgery for grown-up congenital heart patients: survey of 307 consecutive operations from 1991 to 1994. *Am J Cardiol* 1997;80: 906–913). Glancy left a completed manuscript when he returned to the States in October, and Dr. Annie Dore, a French-Canadian cardiology trainee, was left with the task of incorporating the revisions of Somerville. According to Annie, this was not an easy task.

To work at the same hospital with Glancy was a great pleasure, as I had associated with him only rarely in my adulthood. He was the father of my childhood friend, David Glancy, and my childhood memories of him in Maryland and Louisiana were vivid. In August, he invited me to see *Long Day's Journey into Night* by Eugene O'Neill at the Young Vic theater with his younger son, Mark. Having taken a course exclusively on O'Neill at Vanderbilt, I thought I knew something about the playwright until Luke Glancy spoke.

In September, when my father and Lydia Warren, my fiancée, visited London, Luke Glancy invited us to join him and Mark for cocktails at the Barbican residential complex in the city. Glancy had rented a two-bedroom flat on the 36th floor, and the view of London was spectacular. We went on to dine at Vecchio Parioli, an Italian restaurant near the Barbican. During his three-month sabbatical at the RBH, Glancy stayed at this incredible flat and rode the tube for 30 minutes to and from work. Mark Glancy was on the academic faculty of London University, specializing in the history of Hollywood films, those of the 1930s in particular. Several years before, Mark had expressed great disdain for Margaret Thatcher. His dislike of the current conservative Prime Minister, John Major, was equally vehement.

One Saturday, Luke Glancy and I made a "literary walk" through London. His stamina and level of curiosity exceeded mine, despite our age difference. We walked to Bloomsbury and saw the home of Virginia Woolf, then toured The Hospital for Sick Children on Great Ormond Street, before ending up at the bookstores on Charing Cross Road. At the end of his three months in London, Glancy invited all the junior doctors that he associated with at the RBH to an Indian dinner at The Bombay Brasserie on Gloucester Road in South Kensington. It was an act of generosity and friendliness that typified the man.

While on Neville Street those first four months, I was visited, separately, by Lydia and then my father in early September. Born in Mississippi and raised in North Carolina, Lydia had never been north of the Mason-Dixon Line or west of the Mississippi River, let alone to Europe. We had met in Chapel Hill, where she had graduated from UNC. After dating for nearly 2 years, our parting in July was difficult. We so looked forward to her visit in September, which we enjoyed immensely.

I introduced her to Judy and Cyrus Wilson, the Americans, and several other of my new acquaintances. We saw the Jane Austen movie "Emma" with the Wilsons and also saw the play *John Gabriel Borkman,* by Henrik Ibsen, at the Royal National Theatre, starring Paul Scofield and Vanessa Redgrave. On September 10 at the Jurys Kensington Hotel on Queen's Gate, I proposed to Lydia, and she accepted. We could not have been happier, though we had to part again until her next visit in October, when we went to Prague together.

Late in September, my mother Carey Roberts, my sister Frances Roberts, and my mother's companion Bob Berberich visited London. They rented a flat for a week in Earl's Court, which was several blocks from Neville Street. We dined one evening at Nizam, an Indian restaurant, and another at The Bangkok Restaurant off Old Brompton Road. The four of us saw *A Midsummer Night's Dream* at the Barbican the last night, before the threesome left for the Lake District, one of my mother's favorite spots on earth.

Being with my mother in London was like being with an animated British docent with an American southern accent. She would quote Wordsworth, tell us all about the wives of Henry VIII, describe the London life of William Byrd of Westover, give a discourse on Mary Queen of Scots, and explain why "Shakespeare" was the Earl of Oxford. In her book on the Lees of Stratford Hall, she had given the Virginians speech patterns that were right out of Dorset, England. In some ways, my mother took less interest in the 20th century than in the 18th, 17th, and 19th centuries, in that order. I don't think she considered England a foreign country.

It became a pattern that I toured London only when visitors came from the States. By November, I was on call at least two weekends a month, and one of the two weekends, confined to the hospital. The excitement and luster of living abroad gradually settled. The distractions became fewer and the focus became surgery. I had no car, no television, and no radio during the year. I had brought *Cardiac Surgery* by Drs. John W. Kirklin and Brian G. Barratt-Boyes and consulted it regularly throughout the year, especially the chapters on congenital heart disease. In the first few months, I ended each evening with the Kirklin/Barratt-Boyes book, and when I was not reading *Cardiac Surgery,* I generally read Shakespeare.

Chapter 3

Lincoln in Daily Life

For one year, I worked under one surgeon, Mr. Christopher Lincoln. Not only did I learn a great deal *from* him, I also learned a great deal *about* him over the year. Born in England in 1933, the year Hitler came to power in Germany, Lincoln was raised in Kent, the county southeast of London. He spoke only rarely of his parents. When an elderly patient on the ward appeared to be particularly dehydrated, Lincoln would recall how his father had been dehydrated in the convalescent home when he went to visit him. Several times during the year, Lincoln repeated his mother's remark, "It is a mixed marriage, you know," by which she meant a Protestant-Catholic marriage, not an interracial marriage. When he would sew in a patch that was slightly big for the diameter of the heart defect, he would use a simple stitch to gather the patch and make it smaller. Whenever he used that particular technique, he would say, "My mother taught me that."

Lincoln entered medical school at the Royal College of Surgeons and Physicians in Dublin in 1953, the year the heart-lung machine was first used on a patient by Gibbon to repair an atrial septal defect. After the usual six years, he graduated and began a series of "house jobs" in surgery. Four years later, in 1964, he became a "registrar" in surgery and three years later a "senior registrar," in which role he trained for five more years at four hospitals in London: Brompton Hospital, National Heart Hospital, London Chest Hospital, and The Hospital for Sick Children on Great Ormond Street. Apart from these five years of upper-level surgical training, he had one year as a Fulbright Scholar doing research at the Massachusetts General Hospital in Boston. Thus, after a total of 13 years of postgraduate education in surgery, Lincoln was appointed Consultant Cardiothoracic Surgeon at the Brompton Hospital in 1973, at age 39.

As Senior Registrar, he had trained under Paneth and Tubbs at the Brompton, Ross at National Heart Hospital, Sturridge and Belcher at the London Chest, and Aberdeen and Waterston at Great Ormond Street. No doubt he was well prepared for the position in which he found himself in 1973 as a new consultant at the Brompton.

Lincoln wrote his first paper in 1965, at age 32, and he went on to author or co-author some 180 articles by 1998 (see bibliography in Appendix I). During his year at Great Ormond Street, he wrote six papers on congenital heart disease, which would become his subspecialty. Over his 23 years as Consultant at the Brompton, he collaborated with Professor Anderson and Dr. Shinebourne on numerous articles, and their cordial professional and personal relationships spanned this long period.

While his personal manner was eccentric, the consistent theme of his life's work at the RBH was an extremely high standard of patient care. The quality of his surgical care in and out of the operating room was excellent, and he expected excellence from everyone who participated in the care of *his* patients, from his secretary, to the nurse, to the surgical house officer, to the highest level trainee. He published the results of his operations regularly over the years, which is not infrequently a sign of high-quality surgery. The exposure I had to Lincoln's level of quality in cardiac surgery was the greatest education of all, in a year full of broadening experiences.

Certain habits of Lincoln I observed during the year. He never ate during the day. I had never seen anyone do this before, except Nickolas Cokinos, the father of my good friend in Maryland. He, too, ate nothing all day, and then his Sri Lankan servants brought him a feast at night. As I was curious about this dietary technique, I tried it for a week in September. The problem was that I became ravishingly hungry at 3:00 or 4:00 o'clock in the afternoon, to the point of distraction. Certainly it is a matter of habit and discipline, but I chose to discontinue the experiment and resume taking a light, cold lunch at noon.

To sustain his energy, he drank green tea from China. Scallan, the anesthetist, told me that you could trace his movements during the day by following his teacups in the hospital. It was also not unusual for him to stop suddenly in the middle of an operation and say, "I need a cup of tea," at which point a nurse would go to his office, prepare one, and bring it to the operating theater. He would step back from the table, break out of his gown, sip his tea, then rescrub. He said that if he ate breakfast or lunch, he became overcome with inertia; he lacked the energy to go on. During the entire year, I never saw him eat during the day, even as he offered us cake.

Each evening, he drank champagne. He told one of the senior registrars at the RBH, "The only exercise I get is walking down to my cellar every night to get a bottle of champagne." He told me the first thing he did on arriving home nightly was take two aspirin and drink two glasses of champagne. He once commented, "I had just poured my second glass of champagne when I was called to the Wellington last evening to drain a pericardial effusion. You must be fit to do cardiac surgery. Perhaps that is why surgeons retire. It is physically demanding." Not infrequently, toward the end of the day in the operating theater, he would pause and say, "I want champagne." He drank the most expensive Waitrose (British grocery store chain) brand of champagne, which he also routinely served to his guests before dinner. I was never offered bourbon. Lincoln was not an oenophile, and despised what he called "winespeak." He asked Shinebourne to choose the wine at dinner once at the River Café.

Though he ate only once daily, Lincoln took great pleasure in food, the subject of many of our conversations. One morning we talked about the Earl of Sandwich, who created the sandwich that one could easily eat while playing cards. After his return from Brazil, Lincoln remarked that he did not particularly like Brazilian food because it was not prepared to his "European taste." When I was about to return to the States for a brief visit, he asked, "Charles, what is the first food you are going to eat upon your return to the States?" I said I wanted some good vegetables, like corn and lima beans, at Elmo's Diner in Carrboro, North Carolina.

Lincoln had a good reputation for culinary skill. John Simpson, the anesthetist, told me shortly after I arrived in London, "If you ever get an invitation to dine at Christopher Lincoln's home, cancel your invitation to the American Embassy and go. It will be well worth it." Simpson recalled the time that he had invited Lincoln to Christmas dinner. He appeared at Simpson's door with a large Japanese plant and a fresh salmon. After dinner and several bottles of claret, a chauffeur appeared to take him home.

Lincoln's attire and wardrobe were unique. He purchased his typically English, bold-striped shirts at Harvey & Hudson on Jermyn Street. Ties he bought at New & Lingwood. They were of thick, high quality material, not the usual thin silk of Brooks Brothers. A tailor off Old Brompton Road made his suits, though the tailor retired during the year, and Lincoln made inquiries into employing another. He advised me on several points about clothes. He bought only long rise pants fit for wearing braces (suspenders). The pants, he believed, should be unconfining when one sits in a chair. He did not wear a belt, and the pants were not cuffed. He always wore a colored kerchief in his jacket. The color coordination with the shirt and kerchief was sometimes questionable. He had a sizable collection of cuff links, he said, which he kept in a large bowl in his quarters.

When we were preparing to go to Jermyn Street together later in the year, he said, "Charles, reconnoiter Jermyn Street with your father on Friday. Then we will go shopping. I love to spend other people's money. Yes, Charles and I are going shopping." He thought shirts should be tailor-made because the cut is better. One day he appeared at the door and pointed to the sleeves of the shirt he was wearing. "This shirt was bought off the rack. You see the sleeves are too short, as is the tail. The tail of a properly tailored shirt should cover the gluteal region." He said that his weekly dry cleaning bill was about £12 (about 20 dollars). The shirts from Harvey & Hudson were able to withstand years of regular cleanings, he claimed, and when the collar and cuffs became worn, he simply had a new white collar sewn on, and the cuffs turned.

In the locker room at the RBH, he would hang his pants with braces, and shirt with cuff links and tie, on the metal door of his locker, not inside the locker. He never locked his locker; the clothes hung openly in the middle of a row of closed lockers. One always knew when he was in theater. To see patients in the hospital, Lincoln would change into his street clothes. He wore the white coat more regularly than most doctors, always for clinic and formal rounds on Monday and Thursday. To the Wednesday evening grand rounds and to the private hospitals, he wore a suit, as did most consultants.

Lincoln's politics perplexed me. He voted Tory (Conservative) all of his life until March 1997, when, for the first time, he voted Labor. The reputedly unethical behavior of the Tory Party moved him into the Labor camp. Though I did not know the politicians as well as Lincoln, I jokingly expressed concern occasionally about his abandoning the Tory Party. "I'm glad you're not voting here, Charles," he would say to me. I think it was a case of his voting *against* the Tory Party, rather than *for* the Labor Party.

The Tory leader, John Major, was hurt not only by scandals in his own party, but also by differences of opinion over European integration. The fifteen member-states of the European Community were slated to abandon their own currency in favor of a common European currency, to be called the Euro, in 1999. Anxiety was rising over this project in the UK, as well as in Germany and France. "They must hold an election before April," Lincoln said one morning. "This is very exciting." Indeed, Tony Blair won a landslide victory, reclaiming power for the Labor Party after 18 years, with a huge 179-seat House of Commons majority—a greater loss to the Conservatives than Churchill's in 1945.

While Europe was moving toward unity, the UK, paradoxically, was moving toward division, "devolution," as it was called. Scotland, after 290 years of union with England, desired a separate parliament with authority over domestic matters, as did Wales. Neither of these two regions of the UK achieved their goal during my 12 months in London, but it came to pass later in the year of 1997. Like most Englishmen I met, Lincoln expressed no admiration for the Scots or the Welsh, let alone the Northern Irish.

The newspaper Lincoln preferred was the *Financial Times,* particularly the Saturday edition, which he said was "the most informative newspaper in the land." He did not take *The Times* or other daily papers, which he considered too sensational. He also enjoyed reading *Private Eye,* a smaller periodical devoted to ridiculing politicians and unearthing scandals.

One hears that the English always speak of the weather. On a daily basis, upon entering the operating theater, Lincoln would indeed comment on the weather. Lincoln's personality seemed to be affected by it. He had a brighter outlook on clear days. He told my father on his visit that he desired to retire in southern France, where "the weather is good."

Like many Englishmen, Lincoln took an interest in gardening. He grew Japanese maple trees in his narrow backyard, and there was the story that he invited two unsuspecting registrars to his home, then promptly instructed them to prune his trees. In June before I left, his brick-walled garden was lush, like a rain forest.

Lincoln generally held a positive outlook. Now and then he would remark that "between Christmas and New Year's, there is a very high suicide rate. People like me consider it." I don't believe he was particularly religious, though he was respectful of the high church. The evangelical churches he considered lower on the evolutionary ladder.

He told the story of his trip with Paneth, an avowed atheist, to the funeral of a young surgeon in Scotland they both had known. This young surgeon was an evangelistic Christian, and the funeral ceremony was conducted along those lines. Paneth was apparently so put off by the ceremony that he wanted to leave. Lincoln said to me, "You know, it was a church where the minister was always facing *you,* and not the *altar.*" Lincoln added, "A stranger said to me as we were walking out, 'The minister must think we are fools.'" But Lincoln rarely discussed religion.

He did not condone decadent living and slothful ways. He once described a report from the Harvard School of Public Health he had read about 30 years ago. He was so impressed by the report that he got a reprint. The paper described a group of rats that were given all the food they needed, a warm environment, and all the creature comforts. Soon thereafter, the male rats became homosexual, the female rats ignored the male rats, and they all became fat and lost hair. Their society degenerated, because they had nothing to strive for. "It has happened in our society."

Obesity indicated a lack of discipline, in Lincoln's view. Discipline was a word that he used regularly. "Obesity is like cancer," he would say. While common in the States, obesity was relatively rare in the UK. I helped him operate on a morbidly obese patient from Africa at the Wellington Hospital one Saturday morning. The following day, she was seated in a chair and died suddenly, probably from a pulmonary embolism. I shared with him my experience of performing coronary bypass on two morbidly obese patients at UNC. He concurred that operative intervention in such patients probably carries an unacceptable risk of complications.

Lincoln's view of his own country was inconsistent. At times he was extremely proud of British accomplishments, particularly the British Empire. "When England left India in 1948," he said, "India went downhill. If you want to see bureaucracy, go there. The time it took Churchill's soldiers to go by train across India is the same time it takes now." Other times, Lincoln described the UK as "in decline" or "terminal," and his disturbance was obvious.

When an Indian surgeon from Madras came to London to give an address to the Royal College of Surgeons, Lincoln arranged for him to give a morning talk at the RBH. Paul Peters, his senior registrar at the time, was assigned the responsibility of preparing the audiovisual equipment in the conference room, because the surgeon's talk involved a video film of the heart, accompanied by an audiotape. I was beginning an operation and so did not attend, but apparently part of the equipment failed, and the Indian surgeon was forced to deliver his presentation only in part.

Lincoln was furious when he appeared in the operating theater. "We are a third world country," he said several times. "I need to leave this place today as soon as possible." Peters argued briefly that the speaker was late, that he did not come in enough time before the talk to test the equipment. Lincoln countered, "You are never wrong, Mr. Peters." Karen Jurgens, the surgical assistant, and Lincoln had had a disagreement at the operating table the day before, and so Lincoln angrily continued, "Miss Jurgens and Mr. Peters are never wrong, are they, Charles?" No response. "Have you been struck by lightning, Charles?"

Later that day, he was reminded of a headline in one of the newspapers in the UK concerning a catastrophe after a football (soccer) game. Rowdy fans apparently rioted in the streets of one of the English cities, causing great destruction. "Are We a Country of Morons?" was asked on the front page of the local newspaper the next day. Lincoln repeated the question throughout the day.

The day before the audiovisual calamity, Lincoln went with Paul Peters, William Chong, the senior house officer on his team, an Argentine visiting surgeon, and me to the Royal College of Surgeons to hear the man from Madras speak on "The Evolution of the Atrioventricular Valves of the Heart." We walked as a group at dusk on a December day from the RBH to South Kensington Station. As we approached the turnstiles to enter the subway, Lincoln said, looking straight ahead, "Buy my ticket." As we descended on the escalator, he said, "I have not taken public transportation in 20 years."

In the lobby of the Royal College of Surgeons, Lincoln introduced us to Mr. Donald Ross, the distinguished cardiac surgeon originally from South Africa, and his wife, pointing to us individually, "This is Peters, Chong, Roberts . . ." etc.

Lincoln's view of foreign cultures was generally unfavorable. He had the least admiration for the Arab nations. He considered the Arabs desert nomads who had acquired great wealth in the last two generations, the exception being the Omanis, of the southernmost Gulf region. It irritated him that Arabs owned so many beautiful homes in London. He viewed their culture as dichotomous and backward. On one hand, their Islamic religion was morally strict and imposed severe prohibitions on women. On the other hand, the Arabs came to London to play, to free themselves of these religious restrictions. Lincoln said Arab men have literally purchased girls in India as household slaves. "These Indian girls are slaves," he said. ". . . Charles is my slave. An indentured servant." It was toward the end of my year, and we all laughed.

I asked him once if he had received many gifts over the years from patients, and he said, "Generally no, from less than 10% of private patients. Either you receive gifts or you don't. I never did," he said. "In the early days when the Brompton performed heart surgery for Arabia, the gifts were lavish: Rolex watches, cars. There was a male nurse who was a flight attendant for British Airways. Of course they're all homosexuals. He received so many Rolex watches from Arabians he refused to accept any more. He could string them up his arms. . . . I prefer fee for service, no gifts."

Lincoln drove a previously owned Mercedes-Benz in which I rode only once, my second day of work when we went to the Wellington Hospital. During the ride, he described the system of grading architectural structures in London on a scale of 1 to 3. "Mine is grade 2," he said, referring to his home at Pembroke Square in Kensington. I think the chief recreation of Lincoln over the years had been travel. He had been all over the world. During my year in London, he took trips of roughly two weeks' duration to Brazil and to South Africa, always traveling in first class on British Airways.

Chapter 4

Royal Brompton Hospital

A typical day began at 7:30 a.m. with rounds in the Adult Intensive Care Unit (ICU). The registrar (resident) on call in the hospital the previous night was responsible for presenting each surgical patient to the rest of the team. A typical presentation went like this: "Mr. Smith is a 49-year-old who had grafts (coronary artery bypass operation) yesterday by Mr. Pepper. He is on no inotropes, urine is coming, and bleeding has stopped. The plan is to pull his drains and transfer him upstairs." The group then went to the recovery room adjacent to the theater (operating room), where the "fast track" patients convalesced overnight. Patients without major illnesses who underwent routine cardiac operations spent the first postoperative night there, instead of the ICU. The three cardiac teams then separated and saw the rest of their patients individually.

Lincoln's team—the senior registrar, the fellow (CSR), and the senior house officer—musually went to the pediatric ICU next, where two or three patients were seen. We then went to Rose Gallery, which was the pediatric ward, and then up to Alexander Ward, where the adult patients convalesced. In addition to the National Health Service patients, Lincoln sometimes had "private patients," who were cared for on Sir Reginald Wilson Ward, which was specifically designed for such patients. This private ward had its own kitchen, each patient had his or her own room, and each room had a television. After rounds, the Lincoln team went to the locker room, where we changed into blue scrub suits and white shoes and prepared to operate.

Lincoln usually operated Tuesday morning and afternoon, Wednesday afternoon, and Friday morning. Not infrequently, we occupied two operating theaters on Tuesday. We also sometimes operated Wednesday and Thursday mornings. Depending on the need, operations were occasionally performed even on Monday, which Lincoln strongly avoided, because on that day, we organized for the week. After our operations were over each day, the senior registrar, senior house officer, and I went around to see our patients again. By 7:00 p.m., we were usually finished and either went home or stayed in hospital on duty, according to the rotation.

The hospital ICU and wards were in certain ways different from those in which I had worked in the States. The adult ICU at the RBH had four large bay areas, each of which held four patients, one in each corner. In addition, there were four individual rooms off the main hall. The patients were cared for by the surgical team or by a medical team, which consisted of anesthetists and internists. Our surgical patients usually had acute postoperative needs, whereas the medical patients had chronic nonoperative conditions. Patients in the States are usually triaged into physically separate surgical and medical ICUs.

Though the four patients in each bay area were in full view of one another, the nurses kept each patient neatly covered with clean white sheets and blue blankets. This attention to cleanliness and privacy was striking to me in the first few days of work. Whenever a bedside procedure was performed on a patient, the nurse pulled partitions, or curtains on wheels, around the bed.

The adult ICU nurses stayed at the bedside of their patient the entire shift, except for designated breaks when they would arrange temporary coverage by another nurse in the same bay area. I rarely saw more than one nurse at the nurses' station, sometimes no one. This was a major difference in ICU nursing care in the UK and the USA. In the States, nurses often based themselves at the *nurses' station* and went to the patient's bedside as needed. At the RBH, nurses based themselves at the *bedside* and went to the nurses' station only rarely.

Another major difference in ICU care in the UK was the absence of limb restraints on the patients. The typical adult patient at UNC who underwent a cardiac operation had his or her arms restrained by straps around each wrist secured to the side of the bed. The argument was that these arm restraints prevented the patient from personally removing the endotracheal tube or intravascular lines. After appropriate extubation, the restraints were eventually removed. More than one nurse at the RBH specifically asked me, "Is it true that American nurses put restraints on all their ICU patients after cardiac surgery?" Frankly, I had not paid that much attention, until I returned to UNC and found it to be true. In my observation, restraints were never used on postoperative patients at the RBH, which no doubt reflected a more humane approach.

I never saw nurses eating food at or near the nurses' station at the

RBH. Food was eaten in the dining room or behind the closed doors of the break room, which was not even on the ward. This also contrasted sharply with my observation of ICUs in the States, where food was often eaten in view of patients and their families. It should be no surprise that the nurses at the RBH were also, in general, closer to ideal body weight.

Alexander Ward, where adults were transferred for less intensive care, had the same attention to cleanliness and privacy. Every morning, the nurses changed all the white sheets while the patients sat in their chairs eating breakfast. The Alexander Ward also had four bay areas, each holding six patients. Curtains could be drawn around each patient for privacy, and this was done routinely when we examined wounds. One bay area was called a "high dependency unit," in which patients received closer nursing care in their transition from the adult ICU.

One Sunday afternoon on Alexander Ward, I saw six men in the bay area, each in or beside his own bed, quietly reading or resting. It was remarkably peaceful, as there were no televisions or radios permitted on the ward. Though it might strike an American as undesirable to be in a room with five other patients, bay areas had advantages. The men were not isolated during their recovery; one could strike up a conversation with his neighbor. But this arrangement rests on the assumption that each patient is respectful of another's space and quietude. The only time I saw this arrangement in the States was a decade ago at a Veterans Administration Hospital, where the patients were mostly World War II veterans with the respectful manners that characterized that generation.

Our morning and evening rounds were always conducted with a nurse who was specifically assigned to Lincoln's patients. Nurses were either Blue Team (Yacoub and Pepper) or Green Team (Lincoln and Shore/Moat) and were typically well informed about each patient. In the States, the most junior doctor usually presented each patient on rounds, with the respective nurses usually *not* present to offer or obtain information. At the RBH, in contrast, a nurse usually presented each patient to our team of doctors and recorded in a note to herself what the plan was for each patient. These nurses were generally busy and competent.

Patients in the Pediatric ICU and Rose Gallery (the pediatric ward) were under the direct care of pediatricians. The teams of each pediatric heart surgeon (Lincoln, Shore, or Yacoub), however, followed their own patients and intervened when necessary. As in the adult ICU, a nurse was always at the patient's bedside in the pediatric ICU, and the charge nurse, or "sister," supervised.

Each of the three bay areas on Rose Gallery (the pediatric ward) held six children. In addition, four separate single rooms came off the hall. Rose Gallery was Lincoln's least favorite ward. The charge nurse, who was to conduct us through, was often hard to locate or distracted by various ward problems. Rounds in Rose Gallery were usually less organized than elsewhere.

ICU and ward nurses at the RBH wore light blue dresses with a wide, dark blue waistband. The head nurse, or "sister," usually wore a dark blue dress. Only rarely did a nurse wear scrubs outside the operating theater. In general, the nurses were courteous and attentive to patient needs. I did not witness an exchange of harsh words between doctor and nurse. Politeness was the general rule. I was usually called "Charles" by nurses in the ICU and "Dr. Roberts" or "Mr. Roberts" on the ward. In each ICU or ward, one nurse was in charge each shift, and she was actively involved in patient care, always on her feet. The nurses came from many different countries, especially Ireland and Australia. There were others from China, India, Burma, and Mauritius.

The order system for directing the care of a patient to a nurse was different from that in the States. In the adult ICU at the RBH, the doctor simply said, "Please pull the chest drains" or "please pull the neck lines" or "please transfer the patient upstairs," without writing anything. On Alexander Ward, one simply said to a nurse, "Please change the dressing on the leg twice a day," again without writing anything. To prescribe a drug, of course, one did so by writing on a "drug chart" that each patient had at the bedside. The doctor wrote down only drug orders; other orders were given verbally. In the States, what a doctor desires to be done on his or her patient had to be specifically ordered in writing in the patient's chart. A clerk at a nurses station transcribed the order to a patient plan, which was followed by the nurse. This has led to less direct communication between doctor and nurse in the States.

At each bedside, in both the pediatric and adult ICUs, was a computer into which the nurse loaded patient data—heart rate, blood pressure, urine output, output from the chest drains, etc. I was unfamiliar with this system of reviewing patient data—at UNC, such data is recorded on a paper "flow sheet" at the bedside—but I found the computer easy to use and the data neatly arranged on the screen. This bedside computer system was designed by Hewlett-Packard. No misinterpretation of handwriting occurred, and the quantity of paper was certainly reduced. Furthermore, the nurse did not have to leave the bedside to go to the nurses station to write in the notes (chart).

The RBH employed about twenty theater nurses, each assigned to certain operating teams. Vivian Wong, a Chinese woman, was in charge of the Lincoln operating team. A splendid nurse, she was devoted to Lincoln and was one of my favorite nurses. She had several friends in the States, and Francis Ferdinand, the other American fellow trainee, told me that she was quite knowledgeable about the States. Earlier in the year, I had found the round-handled needle holders of Lincoln very slippery, and she made a particular effort to sterilize another needle holder when I was the operating surgeon.

Faye Too was another Chinese nurse who had been at the RBH for many years. Lincoln often used to say while operating with Faye, "You are the best, Faye. Faye is the best." She would occasionally go to his office to make him tea during a long operation. Vivian Wong and Faye Too were devoted and talented theater nurses who had participated in many operations with many consultants and trainees over the years.

Another of my favorite nurses was Dianne Irving, an Afro-Caribbean woman in her twenties who spoke with a Cockney accent. She was extremely kind, and Lincoln would often say to me, "Charles, you need to bring in a tape recorder and record her accent." A main feature of Cockney is that the "t" is silent. For example, better is "be-ha" and Peter is "Pe-ha." Lincoln loved to talk of food and would frequently ask her, "What are you making for dinner tonight?" She sent a nice card and an attractive soap dish as a present for Lydia, my fiancée, and me when we were married in July. Whereas people of color were often called "African-American" in the States, they were called "Afro-Caribbean" in the UK.

Tracy Davies, an English nurse from Birmingham, also frequently worked with Lincoln. Each nurse, of course, had a distinctive style of dressing in the full scrub suit. Tracy wore her hat very low on her forehead, almost covering her eyebrows. I comprehended her strong Birmingham accent better as the year passed. Lincoln once asked three people in the operating theater to say "Birmingham" to compare accents for my benefit. Now and then Tracy would move so quickly that Lincoln would become distracted and say, "Stop moving. You're like a little mouse." Another nurse was from Aukland, New Zealand, from the same hospital as Sir Brian Barratt-Boyes, the distinguished heart surgeon there. When Lincoln first met her in theater, he said jokingly, "Charles, you'd better do the operation. She is from Green Lane Hospital."

Ann Meredith, one of the theater nurses, recommended a hot toddy to me when I was ill with the flu in the dead of winter. Though its effectiveness was unclear, it consisted of whiskey, lemon juice, honey, and hot water. I can still hear her English accent, "hot toddy." As a blond-haired, blue-eyed Englishwoman, she was not unusual in her love of travel. The English and Australian nurses would often visit Africa.

Ann left the RBH in February to live on a tea plantation in Malawi in the lower half of the Dark Continent, for an indefinite period of time. I've known American nurses who desire to visit foreign countries, but not to live abroad.

Nurses were paid very little in London—certainly not enough to live in South Kensington or Chelsea, close to the RBH. To entice nurses to join the staff at the RBH, hospital accommodations were offered at minimal cost, in close proximity to the hospital. As a consequence, nurses came from all over the world to work at the RBH and live in the hospital accommodations. In fact, the accommodations office appeared to give priority to nurses in the choice of flats. The second priority went to senior house officers, because they changed jobs every six months in the various hospitals.

Lincoln was usually patient with theater nurses. He often knew about their lives and would inquire about their child or their boyfriend. In a more humorous mood, he would sometimes ask a nurse to lean over to hold an instrument in the chest, adding "I like your body. Press your body against mine. You won't tell your mother, will you?" Usually when the Chinese nurses returned from their yearly visits to Hong Kong or Malaysia, they would bring him green tea.

For most of the year, the only male theater nurse was Peter Jarin, perhaps the best dressed man at the hospital. His clothes were "bespoke" (tailor-made) and his shoes were always shined. He looked like a banker and, in fact, was a former banker who made a career change into nursing. Lincoln addressed the nurses as "sister" in the operating theater, which was complimentary, in that a sister was equivalent to a head nurse in the States. When Peter operated with us, Lincoln usually kept to his habit of addressing the nurse as "sister," though he would occasionally correct himself and call him "brother."

Apart from the nurses, there was a theater technician called an ODA, which stood for Operating Department Assistant. In addition to the daytime duties, the five ODAs rotated on call at night and were a great help to the anesthetist. They seemed to be principally involved in preparing the anesthetic room, assisting the anesthetist and moving the patient about the operating theater with the porters.

The perfusionists, who managed the heart-lung machine, rotated on call, as well. The perfusionist who worked most frequently with Lincoln was Victor Aston. He was a single Irishman who lived in the hospital accommodations, across the street from the hospital. Adept at operating the heart-lung machine, he was quiet, which suited Lincoln. In fact, he might do an entire case without saying more than three monosyllabic words. This contrasted greatly with the perfusionists in the States, who tended to communicate a great deal with the surgeon and anesthesiologist. Victor was efficient and could assemble and take down the circuit quickly. In the evening, he would return to his room, change clothes, and go to Kavanagh's Irish Pub, under the Jurys Kensington Hotel on Old Brompton Road. There he spent many an evening. Almost every time I went to Kavanagh's during the year, Victor was there, beer in hand.

The demographic characteristics of the staff at the RBH were notable. In general, the "cleaners" (housekeepers) were African, often from Nigeria, the former British colony. They quietly went about their work and would occasionally watch television in the break room. I found two or three Africans watching an American Western movie one Saturday. I occasionally engaged in conversation the Nigerian who cleaned the operating theater. He had been a newspaper reporter in Nigeria, but could not find similar work in London. By the end of the year, however, he had indeed found a job as a London correspondent for a Nigerian newspaper. The porters, in general, were Portugese who kept to themselves. The cooks and cashiers at the cafeteria were primarily from Malaysia, another former British colony. Of the three major races in Malaysia—the Malay, Chinese, and Indian—these were Malays.

Chapter 5

The Surgical Trainees

The senior registrars with whom I worked had been through an educational process somewhat different than that for a chief resident in the States. Rather than four years of college and four years of medical school, the UK doctor went through six years of medical school, consisting of three years of basic sciences and three years of clinical work. At the end of six years, a year of clinical "house jobs" is required before one can be fully registered with the General Medical Council. This year of "house jobs" is similar to the internship in the States, which is required to become licensed. After that, the UK trainee interested in surgery spends three or four years as a house officer before becoming a registrar, then later senior registrar. In the end, the training for a cardiothoracic surgeon after medical school was about ten years, similar to that in the States, if two years of research are included.

The most junior member of the training staff at the RBH was the senior house officer (SHO). In the first four years of training after medical school, SHOs typically changed jobs every six months, in different fields of surgery, usually in different hospitals. SHOs at the RBH were often particularly interested in cardiothoracic surgery and were hoping to gain the support of a consultant, such as Lincoln, in their effort to obtain a registrar position. Though consultant surgeons guided them more or less, the SHOs appeared to have no program director who was responsible for organizing their training or assuring its progress. The SHOs reminded me of "preliminary" general surgical residents in the States who had arranged for only two years or less of training at an institution, rather than the five-year commitment of a "categorical" resident.

The SHOs had varying degrees of surgical experience. They may or may not have had rotations in gastrointestinal surgery, vascular surgery, head and neck surgery, neurosurgery, urology, orthopedic surgery, etc. Many had been in training rotations in cardiothoracic surgery elsewhere and had learned to harvest the greater saphenous vein from the leg for use in coronary bypass operations. Few were capable of good assistance over the heart, however, because they simply had little experience operating.

I came to know five SHOs during the year. The first was Heyman Luckraz, from Mauritius, an island off the coast of east Africa. Mauritius was formerly a British colony, and the ancestors of Luckraz were from India. Heyman and I went to a conference in Liverpool together in late August, my first time outside London. We left the city in a rainstorm on a Thursday night at 10 p.m. I closed my eyes for most of the trip because he drove at an incredible speed in his miniscule sports car. On arrival at 2 a.m. in Liverpool, home of the Beatles, we could not immediately locate the Atlantic Tower Hotel. I spoke with the hotel operator from a telephone booth but was unable to comprehend his speech—the accent was so thick. I learned later that the Liverpool accent is particularly strong, probably derived from the Irish immigrants who came over in the 19th century. Our second night there, Heyman and I walked down to the docks and watched a ferry boat unloading passengers from the Isle of Man.

The conference we attended in Liverpool was held at the Alder Hey Hospital for Children. Entitled "Morphological/Surgical Workshop on Congenital Heart Disease," the course was unique in its concentration of great surgeons and morphologists, way out of proportion to the number of attendees. The faculty included Lincoln, de Leval, and Brawn from the UK, as well as Vouhé and Planché from France. Lincoln clearly admired Planché a great deal. The morphologists included Anderson from London, Becker from Amsterdam, and Thiene from Padua—the European "triumvirate." On Friday evening we dined at The Racquet Club, across from the hotel.

One cold evening in December, Heyman and I went to a typical "curry house" in the east end of London. Heyman ordered a sumptuous meal for us. From the sidewalk, I watched the many Indian cooks through the window after dinner, and they invited me into the kitchen. I stood for a time behind each cook preparing a particular dish. The tandoori oven in which the bread was baked was ingenious.

Heyman showed me the London Hospital, where he attended medical school, and then we went to St. Catherine's Wharf at the Tower Bridge. It was a freezing, windy night, but the sky was clear and the bridge was beautiful. Always polite in daily interactions, Heyman was a tall, slender man with elegant manners. Deborah Sharpe, an American surgical assistant who had lived in London for several years, told me that the Asian Indians whom she knew were devoid of cynicism. This was certainly true for Heyman, who was engaged to a lovely Mauritius woman studying nutrition in London. They invited Lydia and me to their wedding in May in Mauritius, but it was too expensive for us to go.

The second SHO on the Lincoln team in the fall was Chungsen Ko, a Chinese-Malaysian. A rather short, unkempt man whose conversation I usually failed to comprehend, Ko was polite and eventually got a registrar's job at Birmingham through the influence of Lincoln. I always knew when Ko was coming down the hall because he shuffled his feet. In theater one day, when Lincoln remarked that Ko had gotten a registrar's job at Birmingham. I remarked that he needed to stop shuffling his feet, to which Lincoln responded, "Yes, and he needs to buy some black shoes."

Most doctors I worked with, including Lincoln, wore black shoes regularly. Brown shoes or brown suits were rarely worn. I never saw anyone wear that typically American blue blazer, white shirt with tie, and khaki pants. Lincoln and most senior registrars wore suits to work. To wear a tweed jacket and khaki pants to work, as I typically did in the States, was to be casual, almost undignified—dressed for a day in the countryside.

Lincoln and I had several conversations about wardrobe and attire during the year. He firmly believed that one should dress well in the hospital. I saw him only once in the hospital without a tie. It was early in the morning, before we went to theater, and he appeared in the Pediatric ICU to see a sick child. One time on the pediatric ward, he stopped in front of a pediatric registrar who had been on call the previous night. The young man was unshaven and unkempt in appearance. Lincoln pointed to him, saying, "You have not shaven this morning. Charles, this wouldn't happen in North Carolina, would it?" He was under the impression that a strict code of attire was increasingly enforced as one went southward from Boston. This may be partly true. One of the few times I appeared at UNC Hospitals to see patients without wearing a tie, I encountered my chief, Dr. Wilcox, in the hall. He took me aside from the team and told me to wear a tie whenever I saw patients.

The SHOs, registrars, and senior registrars at the RBH also dressed well, in general, perhaps better than their counterparts in the States. American surgical residents often wore scrub suits around the hospital, sometimes going to and from the hospital. This I never saw in the UK. Nor did I ever see running shoes on the feet of surgical trainees ("tennis-shoe doctors"), which had become the norm in the States.

I noticed immediately after arriving in London that the heavy shoes worn by British men and women make a good deal of noise. People walked loudly, even the women. I asked Melanie Cheung, Lincoln's secretary, about this and she said, "Oh yes, you mean clopping." I would walk down a hall at the RBH and hear behind me the sound of a large human being with metal shoes, and yet there would be a lovely, petite, female doctor 20 yards away. It is accepted at all levels of London society, I think, to clop, whereas I recall numerous times in my youth hearing my mother admonish my sister, and even my brothers and me, to walk softly and quietly. The clopping especially resonated at night outside my window on Neville Street.

The third SHO I worked with was William Chung, a married man from Brunei, the extremely small country on the same island as Borneo in southeast Asia. Lincoln had been to Brunei and recalled that the Argentine polo team was visiting the island at the same time. He said that the Sultan, one of the wealthiest persons in the world, flew entire polo teams into Brunei for entertainment. Lincoln had operated on the Sultan's brother's child.

Lincoln remarked that he desired to travel into the Brunei jungle by canoe. "I want to take a canoe inland, no roads. I want to learn how to blow poison darts. It would be very useful here. I can sit in my office and shoot Yacoub or Shore when they pass by my door." The Sultan of Brunei visited London during the period that Chung was on Lincoln's team. Along with other London students from Brunei, Chung was invited by the Sultan to a reception, where each student was handed a brown paper bag containing a substantial sum of money. In theater one day, Lincoln said, "You will mention me, of course, to the Sultan, Mr. Chung." Chung responded, "Yes, of course." "Lincoln . . . L-I-N-C-O-L-N," Lincoln repeated. "Yes, sir," Chung said. "And mention Roberts, too," Lincoln said, at which point I said, "R-O-B-E-R-T-S." Chung sent each of the members of Lincoln's team a Christmas card. He pronounced "three" like "tree," which was not uncommon among Asians speaking English.

In January, the new SHO was Jeremy Prout, a tall, slim, balding Englishman from Somerset. From the very first moment, he was extremely polite. Jeremy was pale in complexion, with thinning hair and long, slender fingers, which he often kept about his face. His affirmative response to a question usually was "Hmm" rather than "Yes." Some Englishmen use this expression regularly in conversation; and others, like Lincoln, rarely at all. At first I was not accustomed to this expression. When Paul Peters, the senior registrar, and I were operating in August, Lincoln poked his head in the door and said, "Put in two drains," to which Peters responded, "Hmm."

Jeremy had occasional physical problems during his seven months on Lincoln's service. He was incapacitated once with a tooth abscess, another time with a gastrointestinal disorder, and another time, he slipped on a waxed floor of the RBH and broke his arm. He smoked cigarettes regularly and had the appearance of one who needed a month of sun, surf, and sand. "A month in Morocco" was what Lincoln advised.

My concern that he would not thrive in heart surgery was shared by Lincoln. Jeremy eventually decided to pursue training in emergency medicine, and Lincoln fully supported him in his successful appointment to a registrar post at St. Mary's Hospital. Lincoln said to me, "St. Mary's is the perfect place for him. He will go far because he is the only surgeon I know who knows what he can and cannot do. Most of us do not admit our limitations."

The physical and mental demands on these SHOs at the RBH appeared to me to be comparatively less than those on surgical residents in their first three years of training in the States, but of course those days for me were a memory, easily embellished. During my first two years of training, for example, I was required to spend every other night at the hospital and rarely left before 5 p.m. on the off-duty evenings. The call schedule for the SHOs at the RBH required in-hospital duty every fourth night. In the States, ward rounds typically started at 6:30 a.m. during my ten years of training—sometimes at 6 a.m. and never after 7 a.m., except on a weekend. At the RBH, rounds always commenced at 7:30 a.m., and the SHO often joined the team 20 minutes later after we left the adult ICU.

The SHOs never "pre-rounded"—that is, saw the patients briefly before rounds to be prepared to present them to the team on rounds. "Pre-rounding" by the junior residents in the States was routine, because the most junior trainee was expected to present each patient on rounds to the chief resident. The SHO at the RBH rarely presented a patient to other members of the team, because that responsibility fell upon the nurse.

During the year I worked primarily with two senior registrars: in the first five months, Paul Peters; in the second half of the year, Anthony Desouza. The final month (July 1997), I worked with Marjan Jahangiri. All three were talented surgeons, each as different as the seasons. Peters, the only Englishman, was the son of a builder (construction worker) from Manchester. He was a bachelor and had started under Lincoln in July, a month before I arrived. During months of laborious negotiations to buy a flat in the Pimlico section of London, Peters house-sat at various places, with most of his possessions in storage. I could reach him only by paging him, as I never knew where he was living. His attire was characterized by the same red tie every day, and then one day he began wearing tweed jackets. At an incredibly low price, Peters had purchased one green and one gray Harris Tweed at a little store in the City. The jackets were handwoven from pure virgin wool in the Outer Hebrides. I later went to this store no less than six times, before settling on one brown and one gray Harris Tweed for me.

Peters gave me two books—one called *Birdsong,* a spectacular historical novel of World War I; and another called *Parkinson's Rules.* I read both, and Lydia later read *Birdsong*. I found Peters to be extremely opinionated, though we disagreed rarely on any medical matter. He was a very knowledgeable surgeon and competent in the operating room.

Over dinner in Prague, Peters quite boldly stated that Americans practiced "third world medicine." I asked him how he arrived at that conclusion, and he said, "Do you remember you told me that you rarely saw rheumatic mitral valve disease at the University of North Carolina? The reason you rarely see rheumatic mitral valve disease is because those patients die at home with their disease, because they don't have insurance to come to the hospital." Of course there may have been a grain of truth to his comment, but only a grain. The main reason I saw so few patients with operative rheumatic valve disease is that antibiotics have virtually eliminated rheumatic fever in the USA. The death rate from rheumatic heart disease per thousand population fell from 7 in 1910 to close to 0 in 1977. Of the roughly 268 million people in the States, about 15% are uninsured. Those who have no insurance are treated when they appear at the door of any state-supported hospital, like Grady Memorial Hospital in Atlanta, or North Carolina Memorial Hospital (UNC) in Chapel Hill.

Peters educated me on one interesting English expression—the two fingers of the right hand held up in the air, in the opposite way that Churchill gave the V for victory. Holding up these two fingers—the forefinger and middle finger of the right hand—means "go to hell" in contemporary use. But the sign is actually a painful reminder to the French of their defeat at the battle of Agincourt, "fought on the day of Crispin Crispian," dramatized by Shakespeare in *Henry V*. The English, according to Shakespeare, were outnumbered five to one, but defeated the French by using crossbows and arrows. Shakespeare wrote that the French lost 10,000 and the English 29. The two English fingers remind the French of the crossbow at Agincourt. I was never at the wrong end of this gesture, fortunately, but I observed its use several times and can confidently say that it is still functional.

Peters, in his relationship with Lincoln, developed a personal rule that I called the Paul Peters Rule. It was his belief that one should neither rejoice when Lincoln compliments, nor fall apart when he criticizes. Peters neither rejoiced nor fell apart during the 5 months I worked with him. Without looking back, I think, Peters returned to the London Chest Hospital in January to continue his training, and from that institution came Anthony Desouza, who went by the name Tony.

Desouza was of Chinese descent, but his country of origin was Malaysia. Though he had little experience in congenital heart disease, he was an extremely talented cardiac surgeon who would have been a superb adult cardiac surgeon *already in practice* in the States. During the six months I worked with him, he performed 69 operations *independently,* under the supervision of Lincoln or another consultant, who did *not* actually scrub in to assist. An American nurse who worked briefly at the RBH claimed he was the best surgeon she had ever seen.

Desouza had a sparkling personality and a contagious laugh. He was always extremely polite to nurses. When asking for an instrument in the operating theater, he would always say "please, thank you" first. For example, he would say, "Forceps, please, thank you," and then the nurse would hand him the forceps. One of his favorite expressions was "bloody hell," and at times he would let loose an unending barrage of American jokes and generalizations, usually delivered with a sense of humor and chock full of inaccuracies. He rode a colorful motorcycle to work each day, wearing his black leather jacket over a dark suit.

One of the most enjoyable aspects of the year was dining out with friends, which I did frequently—Indian food, Chinese food, and Thai food—with great delight. It was during the second six months, however, that I dined out the most, because of my friendship with Tony, who regularly consulted the *Michelin Guide* to London restaurants.

Sarah, his English wife of 6 months, had first trained in oral surgery and then had recently switched to anesthesiology. She was working at the time at St. Mary's Hospital, frequently on call there. Sarah told me that if Tony were not a cardiac surgeon, he would have been a priest or a chef. While he rarely spoke on religion, he obviously knew a good deal about cooking. Most often, we went to the Bayswater area of London above Hyde Park, and ate Chinese food at Mandarin Kitchen Seafood, which served delicious crispy aromatic duck, or the Four Seasons, where we also enjoyed the barbecued duck. We usually let Tony order because he spoke fluent Chinese and seemed to know exactly how much to order.

Everybody liked the aromatic duck, especially Francis Ferdinand, an American trainee, and it always vanished quickly from the plate.

Tony and Sarah Desouza's flat was in Fulham, overlooking the Thames River and the Putney Bridge. They frequently entertained, and it was always a grand culinary experience. Just when one thought one couldn't eat another bite, they would serve dessert. We would sometimes listen to musicals such as "Evita," and Tony would sing the parts he knew. After I returned to the States in July, 1997, the Chinese President Jiang Zemin went to Washington to visit Clinton. I was reminded of Tony because it was said that the Chinese president also sang the Broadway musicals.

One evening after barbecuing on the balcony, Tony brought out the binoculars and we saw a comet in the sky. There was also an unending line of airplanes over their flat, separated by a minute or two, making their approach to Heathrow Airport. The tremendous fluctuation in the tide of the Thames River was remarkable. At 5 p.m., water would be 20 feet from the wall, and at 6 p.m., it would be rising up the wall.

One Sunday over lunch at the Royal China Restaurant in Putney, Desouza gave Ferdinand and me the Chinese outlook on life. He said the Chinese, in general, had no religion and gave no thought to the afterlife. Money was their main interest, apart from their children. They were not interested in politics, and political solidarity among the people was rare. He challenged me to name one Chinese-American politician in the States. Of the roughly 5 percent of Americans of Asian descent, the largest group are the Chinese-Americans. China is a classless society, Tony remarked, in contrast to the UK, and acquisition of money is the major motivation. Despite this characterization, I never sensed that money was a major motivation in Desouza's life. He seemed to be primarily interested in enjoying work with his colleagues. We spent six months working together, which was perhaps my most enjoyable period in my 15 years in medicine.

Marjan Jahangiri replaced Tony Desouza as Lincoln's senior registrar in July. I had the oportunity to work with her nearly four weeks. During the previous six months she had worked at the RBH for Darryl Shore, another consultant surgeon who performed both pediatric and adult cardiac surgery. She clearly had six difficult months with Shore.

Shore was younger than Lincoln and, in fact, Lincoln had trained Shore years before at the RBH. After his first consultant post at South Hampton, Shore came to the RBH, where he was notoriously difficult to work with, if one worked *for* him. Shore always treated me with courtesy, however, and I assisted him on several operations. When I occasionally assisted him on Saturdays, I promptly received a paycheck in the mail, for which I was appreciative.

That Marjan survived the six months proved that she was tough. As Lincoln said, she was like a "terrier." Toward the end of her six months with Shore, Lincoln would say about Marjan, "Two weeks, Charles. All we need is two weeks and she will be back. . . . I will let Marjan gradually increase and you gradually fade out."

Indeed, she seemed to be a new person on Lincoln's service, but I was somewhat surprised at how tough Lincoln was on her. Of the three senior registrars who worked with Lincoln during my 12 months, Tony Desouza clearly got the best treatment, probably because Lincoln felt so comfortable leaving him alone in the operating theater. Tony worked with loose supervision much of the time.

Marjan was Persian, and petite in frame. Before medicine, she had been involved in theater, and I don't mean the operating theater. In that artistic culture she met her husband Jan Latham-Koenig, a musical conductor. His work kept him on the European continent much of the time, while she worked in the London hospitals. While I was in London, he was conductor of the Strasbourg Symphony Orchestra, returning home to London for various periods of time. He was often guest conductor in cities around the world.

Marjan and Jan owned a beautiful townhouse in Chelsea which far exceeded the living standard of her surgical contemporaries in training. She invited Lydia and me, with other guests, for dinner one evening, and it was spectacular. Her home was beautifully furnished, and Lydia and I were introduced to several of her friends in the interior design industry.

One of the mansions on Regent Park had been turned into an interior design exhibition, and several prominent British interior designers had each been given a room in the mansion to decorate. Marjan's Persian friend Alidad, a guest at the dinner party, won the award for the most beautiful room. The day after the party, Lydia and I toured the mansion and found Alidad standing in the corner of his creation, peering at the passersby. His room was a master bedroom fit for a man, a *gentleman*. There was a large, heavy, wooden bed, a fire in the fireplace, a bear rug, a couple of fine old leather chairs on a beautiful Persian rug, and the walls were lined with leather.

All of the guests at Marjan's dinner party had some connection to interior design, and Marjan moved among them easily. She was a sort of super-woman in their eyes—elegant hostess, cardiac surgeon. I did notice one or two servant girls in the kitchen who must have helped Marjan prepare for this evening, as her husband was abroad at the time.

Lydia and I met Marjan and Jan at the Savoy Theatre one evening at a play called *The Importance of Being Oscar,* involving a single actor, Simon Callow, whose performance was excellent. Marjan and Jan were friends with Callow, who was an occasional film actor, as well, with a recent role in "Four Weddings and a Funeral." I had already seen two plays during the year by Oscar Wilde, and this one about his life was poignant.

After the play, the four of us went backstage to see Callow. We were drinking wine in his dressing room when the actor appeared at the door with great vivacity. Callow seemed to be highly intelligent and conversed primarily with Jan about art on a level for which I was unprepared. As I remember, I stood mute, commenting only once that I was familiar with Richard Ellington's biography of Wilde (because Ellington had been a visiting professor at Emory while I was in medical school). Both artists, Jan and Callow, were widely read, and the friction of their minds was scintillating—the conversation moved from music to theater to literature and back.

At the end of July, Marjan and Jan hosted a more informal dinner party in my honor at their townhouse. We sat on the back patio and dined on china at a round table, with candles. When a dog barked next door, Jan's head spun around. He was highly sensitive to his environment—one could see it in the eyes and expression—and I suppose this sensitivity gave him the fine ear for music. The bookshelves in his library contained volumes of music by the great composers, as well as a varied collection of other books. Marjan told me that she had organized the books and music on the shelves. Their home was neat and elegant, and this time, I did not notice servant girls.

I became acquainted with several other registrars or senior registrars during the year. Two Irish surgeons—one in the first six months and one in the second six months—worked with the general thoracic surgical team. Both were Protestants from Northern Ireland, and both were intelligent, affable, and loquacious. Allistair Graham, who worked with Peter Goldstraw the first six months, returned to Belfast in January to continue his training at the Royal Victoria Hospital. He asked me once if most Irish-Americans considered themselves more Irish than American. I responded no. Though Irish-Americans may wear a University of Notre Dame jersey at Saturday afternoon football games, or march in a St. Patrick's Day parade yearly, or even express anti-British sentiments from time to time, the Irish-Americans have not laid down their lives for Ireland, as they have in American wars for 3 centuries, particularly in the last 150 years. In the Civil War, the Union "Irish

Brigade" from New York and the Confederate Irish "Zouaves" from Louisiana were highly respected fighting units. Having never met any Irish-American who expressed a desire to live in Ireland, I believe their Irish loyalty is purely sentimental.

Vincent Young, the other Irishman, worked with the thoracic surgeon Ugo Pasterino, beginning in January. He had been a registrar in Dublin after attending medical school at Trinity University, and came to London at the training level of senior house officer. Over the years, he had worked his way up to senior registrar in the RBH-London Chest Hospital training program. Vincent was incredibly talkative, as they say the Irish are, and had a witty sense of humor. In one of the Oscar Wilde plays I saw during the year, someone remarked, "If only the Irish would speak and the English would listen." Young once said, "I love taking *other* people's patients back for bleeding," which I thought was quite funny. One does feel miserable taking one's own patient back to the operating theater for bleeding, and yet, when the original operation was by a colleague, one feels free of guilt and terribly curious to find the site of bleeding.

Young worked six months with Pastorino, an Italian surgical colleague of Goldstraw. Pastorino was achieving some notoriety as the organizer of The International Registry of Lung Metastases, the updated results of which he presented at a meeting in Dublin that I attended. Pastorino and Young were like oil and water—the Italian and Irish temperaments. Young was waiting patiently to work the next six months with Goldstraw, the older, more distinguished general thoracic surgeon. Goldstraw had employed a Greek trainee named George Ladas, whose Mediterranean temperament had the same effect on Young.

Chapter 6

The Other American

The fellow trainee whom I came to know the best during the year was Francis Ferdinand, from the USA. I liked to kid him about being raised in Newark, New Jersey, a city in decline over the past fifty years. Francis candidly asserted that he was raised on "the wrong side of the tracks," and curiously, was outspoken about the fact that he was educated in Catholic schools, finishing at Essex Catholic High School in Newark. He considered his Catholic school education to be more liberal and broad-minded than the routine American public school education, especially in the area of sex education. Francis won a fencing scholarship to The University of Maryland, where his major was zoology. He also spent a semester in Italy, a sort of sampling of his roots. He took most of his general surgical training at The Medical College of Pennsylvania in Philadelphia, and his cardiothoracic training at The University of Chicago, under Ferguson in thoracic surgery and Karp in cardiac surgery. He had twenty or so publications and was academically oriented.

During his years in Philadelphia, he met Leslie Jeng, a sales representative with Merck. Educated at the University of California at Berkeley, she put her career on hold to come to London with Francis. When Lydia arrived in April, she and Leslie became great friends, fortunately, and the four of us spent much time together.

I enjoyed watching Francis use his hands when he talked, and he spoke articulately. While I brought only three suitcases to London to live for a year, he shipped a great deal of personal effects, including a stack of *National Geographic Magazines* that contained articles on Europe. This was a mark of an inquisitive man, I thought.

While attending The University of Maryland, he had made his first ventures south into the Carolinas to compete in fencing against UNC,

Duke University, and Wake Forest University, which were part of the Atlantic Coast Conference. Evidently, these forays into the South gave shape to his odd opinions about life in the South, which were occasionally irritating. He told and retold the story of how he and his college friends from Maryland were pulled over by a state trooper in North Carolina. On more than one occasion, when describing the Carolinas, he would say to some innocent Englishman, "You know, the people in the South wear the white hoods . . ." One of his surgical mentors in Chicago had married a Southern woman who prepared breakfast for him each morning before work. Francis was convinced that all Southern women were born and bred to so honor and serve their husbands.

Francis and I each took an interest in clothes, motivated, in part, by Lincoln. In January, Lincoln took us to Jermyn Street to shop. After Francis and I purchased shirts, we walked down the street to Paxton & Whitfield, "Cheesemongers since 1797," where Lincoln bought us each a pork pie with mustard relish. Francis seemed to have a good working knowledge of wines and cheeses, ports and different cuisines. I think he dined out even more than Anthony Desouza. One Saturday, Francis and I went again to Jermyn Street to shop and then to The Fountain restaurant of Fortnum & Mason's. We drank the royal blend tea and ate rarebit, which is an open grilled cheese sandwich, more or less.

Francis never refused an offer to dine out. We spent one afternoon at Fileric, a little French café on Old Brompton Road, eating a delicious dessert called flan, drinking cappuccino, and reading the *Herald Tribune* and *USA Today*. On weekends after a busy week, we occasionally spent entire afternoons lounging in his living room or my garden at St. Luke's Street, reading the Sunday paper and snoozing. We could pass the time without a word for hours.

It became a sort of joke with Tony Desouza that Francis would usually fall asleep after one of our big meals, and he always defended his tiredness by saying that he had operated "long and hard" that day, as if the rest of us hadn't! After Tony, Francis, and I lunched at a Chinese restaurant in Putney, we had a three-hour repose in Tony's apartment, sampling various alcoholic beverages. Francis and I then walked the entire way back to Chelsea, stopping in bookstores along the way. That evening at the Picasso Café, we read our books in silence over cappuccino.

One of our most enjoyable experiences was in the room-sized humidor at the Alfred Dunhill store on Jermyn Street. A clerk served us two varieties of single malted Scotch, as we browsed magazines and smoked Cohiba cigars. Francis was a marvelous conversationalist. I rarely went away from him without having learned something. More than one acquaintance of Francis remarked to me that he was a "Renaissance man."

Ferdinand was also a comparative sociologist, as I attempted to be. He made numerous observations on British life, providing an immediate comparison to American life. He also adopted many of the English ways and expressions, such as "Oh, right," which Americans do not say. He easily adopted all the English medical jargon at the RBH. It took me six months to begin saying "theater" instead of "operating room." I think it took Francis six days. Some of his observations on British men and manners were keen. He would point out little particulars that I may have missed; for example, he noted that Lincoln's secretary at the end of a letter typed her name, Melanie Cheung, *followed* by "(Miss)". We compared observations frequently.

Lincoln and I enjoyed talking about Francis at various times. When the three of us were window shopping on Jermyn Street, we stopped in front of a display of shaving apparatus. I remarked that I would like to use shaving soap with a brush at some time in the future. Francis remarked that he already used that method of shaving. Lincoln decided then and there that Francis was a gentleman, "far above" Lincoln and Roberts. He would say, "Charles, I'm surprised Francis even talks to us." The fate of Francis was sealed at Thomas Pink, the shirt store on Jermyn Street, when he bought mother-of-pearl collar stays. He also bought a pair of shoes at Tricker's, the famous old boot makers. The shoes, however, became a painful subject for Francis because they were too small and the leather did not soften as he had expected.

Apart from clothes and food, Francis had several conversational themes that one heard in the course of time. He was particularly angry about tobacco. He regarded it a "drug" that has done far more damage than cocaine, heroine, etc. He also did not like what he considered to be the hypocrisy of feminists. He thought it inconsistent that feminists supported Anita Hill in her sexual harrassment testimony against the Supreme Court nominee Clarence Thomas, and yet feminists seemed to shun Paula Jones, the apparent victim of sexual harassment by President Clinton. Ferdinand also argued that the feminists supported Robert Maplethorpe, the controversial "left wing" photographer of homosexuals, but not Andrew Dice Clay, the controversial "right wing" comedian, whose material was also sexually graphic.

Francis was heavily influenced by the "system" of Dr. Robert Karp at The University of Chicago. His experience in London from a professional standpoint seemed excellent. In particular, he was learning from Sir Magdi Yacoub and Mr. John Pepper how to replace aortic valves with homografts or with Toronto stentless bioprostheses, experiences that would certainly be valuable back in the States. One difference in our training in London was that I was gaining valuable experience in congenital heart surgery, while his was primarily in acquired heart surgery.

Chapter 7

Brompton History

My introduction to the history of the RBH was by Lincoln in August. Our Wednesday clinic was held on the first floor of the South Block building of the Brompton Hospital, which was where Lincoln practiced until 1990, when the new "Royal Brompton Hospital" opened on Sydney Street. According to *The Seven Ages of the Brompton: A Saga of a Hospital,* by P.J. Bishop, B.D.B. Lucas, and B.G.B. Lucas, the original Brompton Hospital in Chelsea in 1842 was called the Manor House, a "hospital for consumption and diseases of the chest." The North Block building of the Brompton Hospital on Fulham Road opened in 1846. Regrettably, the North Block building was being converted to flats during my year in London.

In August, Lincoln gave us a tour of the abandoned building before the conversion to flats began. We entered by crossing under Fulham Road through the tunnel from South Block to North Block. "The Pakistani and Bangladesh servers would push trolleys of food through this tunnel at incredible speed," he said. "They would come around this corner like Ben Hur, spilling custard on the floor." Lincoln also showed us the beautiful interior of Lamb's Chapel, which was part of the North Block hospital.

The South Block building opened in 1882. The operating theaters were on the ground floor, and the ICU was on the very top floor. Lincoln took Peters and me on a tour of these areas. After 1990, the South Block building was used for patients with lung diseases only. When we were walking down the stairs of the old Brompton, Lincoln remarked, "These stairs are composed of half wood and half acid-fast bacilli," which is the bacteria of tuberculosis. All operations, cardiac and lung, were now carried out in the new building on Sydney Street.

On one wall outside the operating theaters in the RBH on Sydney Street was a series of thirteen photographs of prominent Brompton physicians and surgeons. The two major pioneers in thoracic surgery at the Brompton were James Ernest Helm Roberts and Arthur Tudor Edwards. Roberts was surgeon at the Brompton for 28 years, retiring in 1947. Lincoln used a "Roberts clamp" regularly at operation. It was an instrument similar to a "tonsil clamp" in the States, but stronger and heavier. We used it to insert chest drains.

In the first issue of *Thorax* (March 1946), Tudor Edwards published a review of 1,016 cases of bronchial carcinoma, 173 of which he had operated on himself. He died only a few months later. The cumulative thoracic surgical experience of Roberts and Edwards must have been vast. Edwards did a pneumonectomy for bronchiectatic abscess on February 6, 1935; two days later, on February 8, Roberts performed a similar operation. These were the first two successful pneumonectomies performed in the UK. Apparently, extreme rivalry existed between the two surgeons, who were estranged from one another for years.

Henry Philbrick Nelson and Sir Clement Price Thomas were both hired as thoracic surgeons in 1933. Both men had trained under Roberts and Edwards, but Nelson's career was cut short two years later by fatal bacteremia following injury to a finger by a spicule of bone from a rib when draining an empyema. Norman Rupert Barrett and Oswald Sydney Tubbs came to the Brompton as surgeons in 1947, as did Russell Claude Brock.

Brock dominated the early days of cardiac surgery in the UK. Operations on cyanotic congenital heart disease began in Britain in 1947 after a visit by Alfred Blalock of Baltimore, who performed the so-called "Blalock-Taussig shunt." Brock was knighted in 1954 and raised to the peerage as Lord Brock of Wimbledon in 1963. Of all the early cardiac surgeons, Lincoln spoke most often of Lord Brock and Matthew Paneth. To find out more about Brock, Lincoln advised me to interview Ross and Paneth, which, regrettably, I never did.

Lincoln thought it was unfortunate that no one had compiled the aphorisms of Russell Brock. From time to time, Lincoln would repeat some of Brock's sayings, a few of which I recorded. Brock's first major contribution was a book on *The Anatomy of the Bronchial Tree,* which appeared in 1950. In his portrait at the Royal College of Surgeons, in which he is wearing the College robes, Brock is holding a copy of this book. For about six months, Lincoln had a book called *The Life and Work of Sir Astley Cooper* on his desk. It was a biography written by Brock, and I borrowed it from Lincoln and read it during my last week in London.

Lord Brock, who addressed men only by their family name, told the young Lincoln one morning: "I was looking at myself in the mirror this morning, Lincoln, while shaving, wondering which one of my patients today is going to die." Operative mortality in those days was high. Lord Brock also told Lincoln that "you should always, when driving by the hospital, stop in to visit your patients, because one of them will always need you *at that time*." Lincoln found that to be true. Brock told the story once of operating upon a patient when there occurred a sudden explosion. This was during the World War II days of the German air raids. Lord Brock reported to the patient's family, "The explosion you heard, Madam, was not your husband. It was a V2."

Apparently it was Tubbs who persuaded Brock to retire. Tubbs told the aging Brock, "Russell, please stop operating; you are ruining a glorious career." Many of the old Brompton surgeons were described in a book called *The History of Cardiothoracic Surgery,* by Raymond Hurt, a friend of Lincoln. Lincoln kindly bought copies for me and Tony Desouza when the book appeared in 1997.

Lincoln said that Brock saved the old theaters at Guy's Hospital from demolition. The three important medical schools historically in London were St. Bartholomew's, Guy's, and St. Thomas'. I toured only one of these three schools during the year, Guy's Hospital, where Sir Astley Cooper, and later Brock, had worked. Consultants typically had appointments to two hospitals—the Brompton and Guy's, in Brock's case.

Lincoln shared many anecdotes on international figures in cardiac surgery. At the American Heart Association meeting in 1968, he heard René Favalaro, the Argentine surgeon, then working at The Cleveland Clinic, present his results of coronary artery bypass grafting using saphenous veins. Lincoln remembered, "Someone got up and said 'Preposterous' when it was over." At the same meeting, Brian Barratt-Boyes presented results of operations on infants using circulatory arrest. Though he admired Barratt-Boyes as a surgeon and educator, Lincoln once remarked, "To be alone in a room with Barratt-Boyes for an hour . . . what a fate. I do not want to talk about Prolene when I am abroad."

Lincoln commented several times on the history of Prolene suture, "I assisted on the first operation at the Brompton where Prolene was used. It was a coarctation repair. We did a continuous row posteriorly and an interrupted row anteriorly. Postoperatively, the child exsanguinated suddenly. Within a month, a report from Ethicon appeared, stating that five knots must be made with Prolene. We had made only three or four knots—which one needs with silk—not knowing more were necessary." Another time Lincoln remarked "if you're called in the middle of the night that your coarctation patient is suddenly bleeding, turn out the light and turn over in bed. You will never be able to save the child."

Lincoln occasionally repeated the wonderful saying of the surgeon, Sir Berkeley George Andrew, Lord Moynihan of Leeds (1865–1936), "When I need an operation, Oh Lord, save me from the gifted surgeon. Such people should be confined to nimble tricks with billiard balls and bowls of vanishing goldfish." This philosophy was consistent with Lincoln's own approach to surgery, which was simple, straightforward, and safe.

Denton Cooley's name came up one day while Lincoln and I were walking through the old building on South Block. Founder of the famous Texas Heart Institute, Cooley had spent a year with Brock at the Brompton after completing his training at The Johns Hopkins Hospital under Blalock. Cooley's training was quite advanced in closed cardiovascular surgery by the time he started work with Brock. Donald Ross, from South Africa, was Brock's trainee at Guy's Hospital, while Cooley was his trainee at the Brompton. Lincoln remarked that when Tubbs developed tuberculosis and underwent a lobectomy by Brock, Cooley was a Senior Registrar and became a locum Consultant temporarily to replace Tubbs. Lincoln remarked, "I sent Cooley a copy of an operative report signed by him in large handwriting, 'D.A. Cooley.' He replied that he showed it to his residents as an example of a handwritten operative report, in the days before secretaries typed them all." Mark Bleiweis, who entered the cardiothoracic training program at UNC in 1996, had the opportunity to meet Cooley recently, and Bleiweis asked him for advice on where to get an additional "finishing" year of training. Cooley said, "Go abroad."

Chapter 8

Lincoln at Work

The primary purpose of my coming to London was to further my operative experience in congenital heart disease. Lincoln was one of three congenital heart surgeons at the RBH and the busiest there of the three. He had been a consultant congenital heart surgeon for 23 years, and it was a privilege to spend countless hours with him over patients in the operating theater. He was an expressive teacher who made his opinions known. His view of the operative treatment of congenital heart disease was skeptical. In general, he viewed most congenital heart diseases as fatal and believed that resources would probably be better allocated elsewhere. "I think a 65-year-old man with angina pectoris deserves an operation more than an infant with pulmonary atresia and absent pulmonary arteries," he once remarked.

Lincoln did not perform the Norwood operation on children with hypoplastic left heart syndrome (the condition in which the left ventricular chamber of the heart is too small to function properly), because the results were so poor worldwide. These children actually require three operations in stages, and Lincoln chose not to undertake the first. "Any operation whose later goal is a Fontan circulation (procedure) cannot be promising." He believed that when the annals of cardiac surgery are written, we will look back with horror on this period of operating on children with hypoplastic left heart syndrome. Lincoln was not enthusiastic about any operation for single functional ventricle. Francis Fontan, he believed, "has not done the world a good service."

Every Monday and Thursday, Lincoln conducted formal rounds. Angiograms were reviewed and then patients were seen, starting at the top floor on Alexander Ward, where the adults convalesced after intensive care. Before seeing a new patient prior to an operation, Lincoln always reviewed the cardiac angiograms: "Know the anatomy *before* seeing the patient." Typically on his rounds he would try to "do everything at once—see the patient, discuss the operation, obtain consent—so there's no need to come back again." Patient care after surgery he called "housekeeping." It was either good housekeeping or bad housekeeping. Upon gathering at Alexander Ward, we would identify the nurse who knew Lincoln's patients, and she would guide us around. Lincoln would frequently say "Lead on" or "Take me to the patient."

Lincoln spent a fair amount of time looking at the patient, inspecting him or her. He had a remarkable ability to assess the patient's medical status by observation alone. If he was unsure about the patient, he would sit down at the bedside and observe further. Sometimes he would feel the brachial pulse or listen with his stethoscope. He believed that looking at the peri-oral skin color and the color of the hands and feet gave some idea of cardiac output, particularly in children. With one child who was particularly ill postoperatively, he felt the brachial pulse on a daily basis and, in that way, assessed cardiac output. In the pediatric ICU he would often sit down at the bedside and absorb data until he was satisfied that his assessment was accurate and the treatment optimal.

Lincoln was not an advocate of aggressive postoperative activity and exercise. He believed in rest—a slow, easy convalescence, particularly in the elderly. In fact, he thought certain forms of exercise were "unnatural." Running on hard surfaces, he believed, would only lead to premature injury to joints.

He seemed to enjoy interacting with the adult patients the most. As I mentioned earlier, sometimes on rounds he would say, "Charles, listen to his accent. Where do you think he's from?" He liked to pause before a patient and look at him or her carefully in silence. Sometimes he would ask them what their occupation was, and he would take their hand and inspect it, noting the rough hands of a builder. Upon leaving an English woman's bedside, he remarked, "That woman we just saw is a classic example of the typical middle-class English woman. You would find her on Saturday selling jam at her local church."

Once he expressed disdain for the Manchester accent, perhaps not remembering that Mr. Paul Peters, a member of the team, was from Manchester. Peters immediately took exception to Lincoln's remark. Lincoln often asked Tracy Davies, the theater nurse from Birmingham, to repeat sentences in her accent for my benefit. After bringing to my attention the accent of a man from Kent, Lincoln said that in the spring the poor from East London would sometimes spend "working holidays" in the hop fields in Kent. Groups of families would stay in a village together, and one would hear the Cockney accent of the East Londoners in the Kentish pubs.

If a television set was on when he entered the room, Lincoln would invariably say, "Turn the box off. Turn the box off. It rots the brain." He usually fiddled with the dials in trying to turn it off because he was so unfamiliar with televisions. He remarked several times over the year, "I detest television."

In a room at the end of the children's ward, a "school" was held regularly for pediatric patients. We had to walk by the room daily, and Lincoln would often stop at the door and watch the children. While observing the teachers and students, he expressed no emotion, except once. One Thursday afternoon, we approached the room and heard the clamor of instruments. At the door we watched about six adults and six children playing various instruments in concert, with great earnestness in this small room. There was a violin, a cello, a guitar, a piano, and two or three strange instruments—one child was smashing a spoon against a serrated wooden board, something one might see played in the French Quarter in New Orleans. The whole musical ensemble, however, struck me as something one might witness on a porch in Appalachia on a summer night. Lincoln and I enjoyed this scene so thoroughly, we laughed heartily over it for days. We were told later that several of the adults in the musical group were from the London Symphony Orchestra, kindly volunteering their time.

One little English child on the ward reminded me of "the Artful Dodger" in *Oliver Twist.* He expressed himself with great enthusiasm and confidence on the telephone at the nurses station. Another child reminded me of Oliver Twist himself. English children in general were very polite when we came to see them. They complained very little, and the nurses frequently complimented them by calling them "brave." A certificate of "bravery" was posted above their bed after they underwent operation. The term is seldom used in the States.

Lincoln did not enjoy answering the endless questions sometimes posed by foreign patients and their families on the private ward. An Indian patient and his family subjected him to a barrage of questions one afternoon, which Lincoln characterized as "a reflection of distrust." He remarked that "the farther you are from the equator, the more trust, the fewer questions. Maybe we trust too much." Lincoln had little patience for nagging, unintelligent questions posed by poorly educated parents and patients. He would usually answer with short monosyllabic responses. He certainly would not respond with long, elaborate descriptions of an operation, because he believed it would make matters worse; it would increase, not decrease, their terror. Desouza told me that Lincoln told the questioning parents of one child on whom he was planning to operate, "It has taken me ten years to understand this operation. I cannot explain it to you in ten minutes."

When meeting an adult he planned to operate on the next day, Lincoln would introduce himself in the following way: "How do you do, Mr. Jones. I'm Mr. Lincoln, the surgeon. I plan to operate on your heart tomorrow. Do you have any questions?" Most patients had no questions, conversed politely, and would agreeably sign the consent form. When patients did have questions, Lincoln's answers were courteous and brief.

The more challenging interviews came on the pediatric ward, with the parents of children who were to undergo an operation. He would ask the parents to leave their child in the crib and then come with him to a separate office at the nurses station, where he would discuss the operation in a quiet setting. A typical interview went as follows: "I'm Mr. Lincoln, the surgeon, and I plan to close the hole in your child's heart tomorrow. There is a risk to the operation, and by 'risk,' I mean the risk of death. There is also a risk of injury to other organs of the body, such as the brain and the lungs and the kidneys. Though it is highly unlikely that this will happen, I must tell you, and I am telling you in the presence of these people here, who will record in the notes (chart) that I am telling you." After answering any questions, Lincoln would say, "Well, then, if you agree, please sign here," handing them the consent form. After this, Lincoln would often remark, "I have nothing more to say. Thank you very much." Most Americans, I suspect, might perceive the interview as cold and hard. It was Lincoln's way; he expressed no insincere concern or emotion. I have seen American surgeons, in their desire to be liked, overcommunicate information to patients and show concern which was not genuine. Lincoln's approach was refreshingly to the point.

I was told one story about Lincoln seeing an elderly woman for a heart operation the next day. She told him that she was very anxious, that tomorrow was one of the most important days of her life. Lincoln calmly responded that he was *not* anxious and that tomorrow was *not* a particularly important day of his life. After Lincoln left the room, she told his assistant that she found his comment strangely comforting.

After rounds on Monday afternoon, we often met in Lincoln's office for cake. Melanie would help us to tea or coffee as we sat around his desk. Lincoln usually bought a cake at a bakery near the Wellington Hospital, where he spent Monday mornings after the RBH conference. Lincoln never ate any cake, but did not seem to mind when we indulged.

He kept a teapot on the floor of his office and would prepare his green tea. On these Monday afternoons, the conversation would range from the surgical methods of de Leval to the quality of the Brazilian beaches.

Early in the year, Lincoln made it clear to Peters and me that we were not permitted to loiter about his secretary's office. Melanie was a beautiful, talented woman in her twenties who was the most efficient secretary I have seen. I reminded Lincoln now and then that he was most fortunate to employ her. Of course he knew that and, in fact, I think he was somewhat territorial about her. He did not want us in her office unless our interaction was brief and strictly business.

Lincoln's skeptical view of his colleagues at the RBH was not unexpected, given his 23-year consultant career there. "All the recently hired consultants are lightweights," he once said, and I think his general view was that the consultants of old were a more formidable group. He did not mingle with other surgeons at the RBH, and rarely had anything positive to say about them.

The anesthetist he worked with the most was Michael Scallan. Originally from South Africa, Scallan was incredibly efficient in the operating theater. He spoke rarely and quietly, and was technically superb at placing intraarterial catheters in babies. He would also join Lincoln in the private sector at the Wellington Hospital or Harley Street Clinic. When I assisted Lincoln at one of these hospitals, Scallan would usually give me a ride there from the RBH. He was expert in both pediatric and adult cardiac anesthesia.

Lincoln would sometimes instruct an anesthesia registrar on some point. When Scallan re-entered the room, Lincoln would say, "Dr. Scallan, I am teaching your registrar cardiac anesthesia again." Later in the day, Scallan would always counter that he had to teach one of Lincoln's registrars something. Scallan liked efficient operating as much as Lincoln. If ever one paused toward the end of an operation, Scallan would peer over the ether screen: "Don't stop. There is always something to do."

Lincoln did not like chatter in the operating theater, especially whispering. If anyone struck up a conversation in a whispered tone, Lincoln would stop operating and ask, "Is something wrong?" In the London buses, there was a sign beside the driver which said, "Do not speak to or distract the attention of the driver when the bus is moving." Lincoln would occasionally quote it. The operating theaters at the RBH were, in general, much quieter than those at UNC. The nurses spoke softly and rarely, the perfusionists answered in monosyllabic words, and the anesthetists tended quietly to their business. In this serene scene, Lincoln did his work.

Lincoln's operative approach in congenital heart cases was educational to watch. He had rather large hands and fingers, and their movements were careful and deliberate. Wasted movements were rare. He once said, "Charles, if my hands were smaller, I would be a great surgeon." He was a "fast" surgeon by the criterion that the operations were completed quickly, but to watch him, one would not call him fast. It was by doing things correctly the first time and eliminating unnecessary moves that time was saved. Most people who watched him operate came away very impressed with his technique. My chief at home, Dr. Wilcox, remarked that he had not seen "a better congenital heart surgeon than Lincoln."

The pediatrician with whom Lincoln had the most interaction was Elliot Shinebourne, who referred most of his patients to Lincoln. Shinebourne came to the RBH just a year before Lincoln and was instrumental in recruiting Lincoln, then a senior registrar at The Hospital for Sick Children on Great Ormond Street. Their relationship spanned over 25 years, and they treated each other with respect and courtesy. The other cardiologist that Lincoln appeared to admire and whose opinion he regularly sought was Derek Gibson. All the adult patients who were to undergo a valve operation were sent to Gibson for an echocardiogram. He was a bachelor who lived in Chelsea, and Lincoln would say, "You can set your watch by him in the morning. He will appear on King's Road at ten minutes to eight."

Lincoln usually came to work on Saturday and Sunday, if only briefly, and would usually see several patients, especially those who were critically ill. I sometimes ran into him in the hall and occasionally found him alone in his office, no one else there on the entire hall. One Sunday in his office he explained to me how "honours" are bestowed by the monarchy twice yearly—Lord Brock was a Life Peer, and Sir Magdi Yacoub was a Knights Bachelor, neither of which were hereditary honours. We went through the various orders of the Companions of Honour, of the Bath of St. Michael and St. George, and of the British Empire. This form of recognition by the government struck me as admirable. The USA also marks people of distinction, but society emphasizes egalitarianism and really accepts no elitism, which is what these British Honours promote.

The senior registrar and I alternated in taking call *specifically* for Lincoln's patients throughout the year. We each took the formal hospital call as well, but considered that a separate duty. After a full day of operating on children, one of us would usually stay until 11 p.m. or so in the evening to watch over the children. Although they were cared for primarily by the pediatricians, Lincoln insisted that we follow them closely. He would regularly call at 8 p.m. and sometimes again at 11 p.m., to check on their status.

Lincoln was realistic in terms of their outcome. We lost four children during the entire year, and it was always fairly clear to him who would not survive. Out of ten arterial switch operations that he performed during the year, one child died. The intraoperative course was stormy, and postoperatively the child was on multiple drugs. At about midnight, I went home; and just as I stepped into my flat, I was called back to the hospital because the child had suddenly arrested. Within minutes, I was in the pediatric ICU and opened the child's chest. The heart was absolutely flaccid and noncontractile. Efforts to restore a heart rhythm and beat were futile, and I called Lincoln to tell him as much. He said, "Oh no, no, no, no, no. That heart will not come back. Thank you." And the conversation ended. As is typical after the unfortunate death of a patient, Lincoln was solemn for a period of time until the work brought him out of it again.

Chapter 9

Monday Morning Conference

The Monday morning conference at 8 a.m. at the RBH was devoted exclusively to children with congenital heart disease. Shore's patients were routinely presented first, because Monday was one of his operating days and they had to get on with their morning case. Next, a member from Lincoln's team presented Lincoln's patients for the week. I alternated with the senior registrar on Lincoln's team in presenting. Usually four congenital patients per week were operated upon by Lincoln. After the patient data had been presented and the echocardiogram or angiogram reviewed, a brief discussion followed.

In Lincoln's view, the main purpose of the conference was for minds to meet to ensure that a consensus was formed regarding the operative procedure planned. It was time for the final decision. Lincoln always sat on the extreme front right, usually sipping a cup of tea. He usually came into conference directly from his car, wearing a suit and carrying his briefcase. Shinebourne sat somewhere to his left, and Michael Rigby, another pediatric cardiologist, always appeared about ten minutes late, joining them on the front row very slowly and deliberately. Professor Robert Anderson, the cardiac morphologist, also sat regularly on the front row, and his presence guaranteed a debate of some sort. Standing in the back were Shore and Professor Andrew Redington, a young pediatric cardiologist. Redington regularly referred his patients to Shore, though not always. Lincoln found it somewhat irritating that Shore and Redington stood in the very back of the room, rather than joining the others in the front.

Manjit Josen was the echocardiographic technician. He usually presented the echocardiograms on each patient and did so in a spectacular way. I remember Lincoln said to Manjit during a pause, "Carry on. I like to hear you talk."

Lincoln could always be counted on for a humorous comment at least once a week. When Rigby was discussing a patient from Greece, he mentioned that the child's transportation to the UK and the bureaucratic paperwork involved was much easier now that Greece was in the EEC (European Economic Community). Lincoln perked up and asked, "Is Harefield in the EEC?", with special reference to his rival, Sir Magdi Yacoub, the internationally known surgeon at Harefield Hospital who operated on patients referred from around the world.

Once, when a particularly challenging patient was discussed at conference, Lincoln remarked, "See him in six months in outpatient clinic . . . . That is our classic delaying tactic. By then, we will have gathered more courage, more clarity of thought." Lincoln walked in conference one day and pointed to an attractive woman two rows back and said, "There is a Brazilian," and then sat down. He never failed to notice a beautiful woman. "Who is that lovely girl?" he would sometimes say in the theater, as he gazed at the beautiful eyes of a woman visitor, otherwise covered by a gown, bouffant, and face mask.

Professor Redington was particularly expert in percutaneous interventional cardiologic procedures, and Lincoln now and then would make comments such as, "Where do you learn these tricks?" The coil occlusion technique for patent ductus arteriosus particularly irritated Lincoln. I think Lincoln was correct when he said that a young congenital heart surgeon at the RBH would have to be extremely firm. It was not infrequent that the spectacular results of Frank Hanley, a pediatric cardiac surgeon at the University of California at San Francisco, were discussed, with the implication that such spectacular results were easily achievable at the RBH. Lincoln's results were superb, even on difficult cases, and he published his results over the years in numerous articles; but he chose not to make a regular practice of performing "fantastic" operations, as he put it.

Chapter 10

Wednesday Grand Rounds

The venue of the Wednesday evening Grand Rounds was the Paul Wood Lecture Theatre at the National Heart and Lung Institute on Dovehouse Street, one block from the RBH. All the physicians and surgeons appeared in dark suits, while the trainees usually wore white coats. The Grand Rounds were conducted by Derek Gibson, the distinguished cardiologist who specialized in echocardiography. Gibson and Lincoln always sat on the third row, with no one in the first two rows.

Gibson was a bibliophile who frequently went to Harrington Brothers Bookstore on King's Road. He referred to Harrington Brothers as "my bookbinder." I asked him once what were his particular interests outside of medicine, and he replied "15th and 16th century architecture. There are only two things to see in London: the Soane Museum (near Lincoln Inn Fields), and the Dulwich Art Gallery." He admired Boswell, whom I was reading at the time, particularly his London journals. The British historian Macaulay came up in conversation, and Gibson dismissed him, then proceeded to quote a page from an essay by Macaulay on the Roman Catholic Church. Gibson believed that the Earl of Salisbury was "the most intelligent prime minister of Great Britain in 200 years." I frequently saw Gibson walking along King's Road in Chelsea.

Lincoln was fond of recalling the conclusions of an outside review panel for the RBH several years ago which found Derek Gibson "unnecessary." Lincoln admired Gibson's mind and said, "He is wasted in medicine, keeping old crocks alive." Gibson funded his fellows apparently with "soft money," like Lincoln, who also told me Gibson refused the distinction of Professor of Medicine at Imperial College, regarding that title with such reverence that he felt himself unqualified. Criteria to become Professor in the UK had fallen, but not nearly so low as in the

States, where it is simply the last step on the standard academic ladder. Gibson told me that he was working in the ICU when the first patient who underwent a Ross operation (aortic valve replacement using a pulmonary homograft) by Ross rolled in from theater.

I said "Good morning" to Gibson one day, and he replied, "Is it?" At Grand Rounds, Gibson would destroy anyone who made an unintelligent comment, or even an intelligent comment, if he disagreed. He believed that the transthoracic method of echocardiography was as good diagnostically as the transesophageal method for any cardiovascular disease. As I mentioned earlier, Lincoln wanted all his valve patients evaluated by Gibson, and Lincoln specifically instructed the trainees to fill out the request form in proper detail, so Gibson would know what to look for. I asked Gibson what kind of substitute valve he would prefer if his aortic valve needed replacement, and he said a homograft, a human valve from a cadaver which is preserved by freezing it.

At the Wednesday night Grand Rounds, two presentations were typically given, and these presentations were assigned months in advance. Typically, Lincoln's team gave one presentation every six months. I was assigned to give a presentation in late October, and Lincoln chose as a topic a challenging patient with congenital heart disease.

The child we operated on was three years and ten months old and was born with a left ventricular chamber that was minute in size. Effectively, the child had only one ventricle, which was the right ventricle, and it pumped blood to both the lungs and the body. Consequently, there was a mixing of red, oxygenated blood with blue, unoxygenated blood. Normally, red blood is separated from blue blood; the circuit is "in series" rather than "in parallel." In the operative treatment of children with a single dominant ventricle, the approach is usually to bypass the heart and channel the blue blood (venous blood) directly to the lungs, where it is oxygenated. This requires creating a pathway either through the heart or around the heart, using baffles or tubes. Our child underwent such a procedure, and it required special considerations because the blood return *from* the lungs was also abnormal. Normally, blood returns to the left atrium (left upper chamber of the heart), but in this child it returned to the right atrium (right upper chamber). Therefore, in making our channel for blue blood to go to the lungs, we had to bypass the entire heart, rather than place the channel through the right atrium, which would obstruct the return of blood from the lungs.

The operation went extremely well, and the child recovered well. We took photographs at the operation and also had a medical illustrator draw a picture of the final result, based on our sketches. I reviewed the literature thoroughly and prepared intensely for this presentation. On the day of the presentation, I mastered all the audiovisual equipment in this large auditorium so that the flow of the presentation would not be impeded. Much to my delight, the presentation went well. The operation and concepts appeared to be understood by much of the audience. Lincoln described the presentation as "perfect," and this certainly made the effort worthwhile. His team was "on stage" before his colleagues only once every six months, and so I understood the importance he attached to such presentations.

We decided to report the patient in an article, which was later published in the *Journal of Thoracic and Cardiovascular Surgery* (see Appendix III). The idea for the operation originally came from Marc de Leval, a congenital heart surgeon at The Hospital for Sick Children on Great Ormond Street in London. When returning from the meeting in Liverpool in August, Lincoln had sat beside de Leval on the train. "I had a fruitful ride with de Leval. He said he has abandoned his own total cavopulmonary connection (which he devised) for an extracardiac conduit. He thinks laminar flow is superior in the extracardiac conduit." It was this serendipitous meeting on a train that stimulated Lincoln to perform this particular operation in the Greek child. Lincoln often described de Leval as "a philosopher," and would occasionally remark on his "weekly call" to de Leval for his surgical opinion. Lincoln's desire to do the right thing for the patient, if necessary to seek another opinion, was admirable. Lincoln believed that when this era is described in the annals of cardiac surgery, de Leval will be described as Britain's best congenital heart surgeon.

Over the years, I had heard my father mention Jane Somerville several times. She was a pediatrician who specialized in congenital heart disease in adults, a subspecialty she virtually created. First at the National Heart Hospital and then at the RBH, her unit was called GUCH, which stood for "grown-up congenital heart" patients. These patients were perhaps the most complicated and difficult cases to manage of all patients with heart disease. They had usually survived operations for their congenital heart malformations, but now suffered persistent complications. Somerville had trained several people in the world in this particular area, including Carol Warnes, who also spent two years with my father at the National Institutes of Health. Warnes had established a similar unit at the Mayo Clinic.

Lincoln had known Jane Somerville for 30 years, since 1966, "and I assure you she hasn't changed," he said, remarking that "she saw herself as the next Helen Taussig," the famous pediatric cardiologist at The

Johns Hopkins Hospital a generation earlier. Somerville usually referred her patients to Professor Yacoub, and so I rarely interacted with her during the year. She was undoubtedly a wonderful speaker and a clear thinker. Lincoln remarked that she had taken a special course in public speaking early in her career. She was married to Walter Somerville, an older, distinguished cardiologist, who was for many years editor of the *British Heart Journal*. During one discussion after a presentation at grand rounds, Somerville got into a spirited repartee with Lincoln about the Fontan operation. One could detect no animosity; in fact, there was considerable humor on both sides.

Lincoln said on more than one occasion, however, that "young surgeons should avoid her. She has ruined many a surgeon's career—I don't mean consultants, I mean registrars." Lincoln pointed to me and said, "Charles, she might be at a meeting in the United States and a registrar's name might come up. She might say, 'Yes, I know Mr. Carter. A nice young man. (Long pause) He still has a lot to learn,' which is the sort of simple comment that can have disastrous effects. That is why, whenever I am asked by non-surgeons how a young surgeon is coming along, I reply favorably, to avoid this kind of disparaging effect."

Chapter 11

Park Walk

At Thanksgiving in late November, I returned home for a brief visit. It was my first time back to the States in four months, and I went first to Chapel Hill to see Lydia. It was a wonderful reunion with my fiancée. We made plans for her move to London in the Spring. We also saw the movie "The English Patient" during my visit, which was superb. The Varsity Theater in Chapel Hill was so filled that we had to sit separately. The movie came to London in January and was a sensation in the UK. *The Times* of London described it on New Year's Day as the best movie of the coming year.

I then flew to Nashville, Tennessee, picked up my daughters Amelia and Camille, then flew to Dallas, Texas, with them to stay with my father ("Granddaddy" to the little girls). We had dinner at his favorite French restaurant, Chez Gerrard, and went the next day to the home of Dr. and Mrs. Robert Kramer for Thanksgiving dinner, with Lydia, who arrived that morning from Chapel Hill. The usual Washington Redskins-Dallas Cowboys football game was on television. We also dined at the Crescent Club and, the last night, at The Old Warsaw. Camille, becoming sleepy, put her head on the white tablecloth at one point and said, "Daddy, why do we have to go to these fancy restaurants? Why can't I just have a hot dog?"

Upon my return to London, I moved to 57 Park Walk. Cyrus and Judy Wilson, my American friends, had decided to spend six weeks in the States and offered to let me stay in their home during that period. It was a wonderful opportunity to live rent free in a three-story townhouse full of creature comforts. The bed was comfortable and the living room was plush, with a television and music system. The kitchen also was clean and well stocked.

Park Walk was about six blocks west on King's Road from Sydney Street, which meant a longer walk, so I left at 7:10, rather than 7:20 a.m. If I were to break the year up into "streets," I came to know Old Brompton Road while living on Neville Street, Fulham Road while living on Park Walk, and King's Road while living on St. Luke's Street. These were the three major streets that ran parallel in Chelsea and South Kensington. I was occasionally teased later in the year that I never left SW3, the postal zip code for South Kensington and Chelsea.

Reading occupied a good deal of my time during the fall on Neville Street, and it continued on Park Walk. While living on Neville Street, I read three Shakespearean plays: *Henry V, Richard III,* and *The Tempest.* The momentum in drama waned, however, and I moved on to the great Samuel Johnson upon arrival at Park Walk. He was a monumental discovery for me. In a little rare book store in Chelsea, I found a Library of Classics edition of *The Life of Samuel Johnson,* by James Boswell, nicely bound in green. Though a pocket-sized, abridged edition, it still ran to 637 pages. I derived immense pleasure from this volume by Boswell. Johnson was the most important literary figure in England in the 18th century, and Boswell introduced me to his English mind. Of course Johnson despised American colonists who gained their independence during his lifetime, but that was no matter. Reading about Johnson brought on wonder and excitement similar to what I had experienced when reading Ezra Pound for the first time 15 years earlier.

Born in Litchfield, Staffordshire, the son of a bookseller, Johnson spent three years at Oxford, leaving without a degree. At age 28, he went to London, and a year later published his first important poem, "Imitation of Juvinal's Third Satire." In 1755 at age 46, he published his greatest work, a *Dictionary of the English Language.* It was a testament to his genius and self-education. Eight years later, he met Boswell, who ensured his literary immortality.

After reading *The Life of Samuel Johnson* in an abridged form, I read much of the *Selected Writings of Samuel Johnson.* For two weeks, I carried around *The Sayings of Dr. Johnson,* edited by Brenda O'Casey; during the last two months, I read a lighter book by Hesketh Pearson, entitled *Johnson and Boswell: The Story of Their Lives.* One of the most exciting afternoons was spent later in the spring at Dr. Johnson's house at 17 Gough Square in the City. It was there that Johnson worked for many years to compile his Dictionary, and where he formed that nucleus of friends which included the painter Joshua Reynolds, the actor David Garrick, the philosopher Edmund Burke, and the writer Oliver Goldsmith. I gave Lincoln a copy of Boswell's biography of Johnson upon my leaving London, with the hope that in retirement in the south of France he might enjoy it as much as I have.

Other random books during the year caught my interest: *Ezra Pound in Kensington* by Hutchins, *Memories and Essays* by Allen Tate, *The Conquest of Gaul* by Caesar, *History and the Reader* by Trevelyan, *The Historical Figure of Jesus* by Sanders, *D. H. Lawrence* by Richard Aldington, and *The Table Talk of W. H. Auden* by Alan Ansen.

Caesar's description of the Gallic and Germanic characters was interesting. Those west of the Rhine were brave and impetuous but lacking in steadiness and perseverance. They were superstitious, and Mercury was the god they most revered. The Gauls gradually became accustomed to inferiority and defeat in battle, however. They did not even pretend to compete with the Germans in bravery. Those east of the Rhine were Barbarians, pursuing hunting and war, not agriculture. They lived on meat and milk and cheese, and worshiped the Sun and Moon and Fire. The word "honor" was often on the lips of Caesar.

During the Christmas season, there were numerous parties, and I attended one in particular sponsored by the theater nurses, held at Cafe Lazeez on Old Brompton Road. It was a sit-down dinner of four tables of operating theater personnel. One humorous scene occurred when Yacoub telephoned Lincoln by a portable phone at the table to encourage him to join us. Apparently Lincoln refused, as he did not typically attend such parties.

One of Lincoln's former senior registrars, who finished just before I arrived, was a Pakistani named Haznat Khan. We lived next to one another, in the front apartments of 18 and 19 Neville Street, respectively, and so I came to know him early in the summer. Two prostitutes lived in the basement flat below him, and the police were occasionally knocking on Haznat's door to inquire about them. After working with Lincoln at the RBH, he went to work with Yacoub at Harefield to complete his doctorate. He had a delightful personality, with sparkling eyes and a keen wit. He seemed to spend many evenings with Victor Aston, one of the cardiac perfusionists at the RBH. A few times during the summer and Fall, I went to Kavanagh's Irish Pub below the Jurys Kensington Hotel on Old Brompton Road, and found Haznat and Victor there, sipping the golden ale.

During the fall, much publicity arose about Haznat Khan in the tabloid newspapers concerning his reputed relationship with Lady Diana. Evidently, Lady Diana had a friend who underwent an operation at the RBH, and she went there regularly to visit. Khan met her at the hospital and they became friends. I know not precisely what their relationship came to, but he had certainly achieved celebrity status by Christmas. Whenever he appeared at one of these hospital parties or an afterwork pub gathering, the women from the hospital who knew him would swarm him. The less he said about his relationship with Lady Diana, the more his celebrity rose.

Haznat appeared in a feature article in a major London tabloid newspaper at least once a week during the year. On May 25, 1997, for example, there appeared on page 3 of the Sunday *Mirror* an article headlined, “Anything Di Khan do, I Khan do better . . .” One amazing circumstance occurred in July when a reporter appeared at the door of Lincoln’s home in Pembroke Square, in search of Karen Jurgens, the surgical assistant and friend of Lincoln. This paparazzo had recently photographed Haznat with his arm casually around Karen at the Wesley Arms Pub, across the street from the RBH. Ignited by the thought that Haznat might be seeing another woman besides Lady Diana, the photojournalist pursued Karen at Lincoln’s home, but to no avail.

I saw Lady Diana when she came unannounced one day to the RBH. As I stepped into the elevator, there she was in the front beside the wall, facing the door with her eyes averted to the wall, a slightly downward gaze. No one was with her, and the Portugese porter in the elevator was nonchalant. She was taller than I expected with a womanly, not too slender, frame. Later that day I passed her walking with an elderly patient in the hall, his arm holding onto her shoulder.

Lincoln told me that the locks on the doors of the two pediatric wards were placed because Lady Diana would appear unexpectedly on the ward in the middle of the night to visit the children. He said that when Lady Diana appeared at the RBH, everyone went on in a British sort of way as if nothing unusual was happening. She was paid no special attention by the hospital staff.

There was a photograph on the pediatric ward of Lincoln in his white coat walking with Queen Elizabeth II and her entourage toward a child. But Lincoln had no high regard for the current generation of the royal family. He seemed to dislike Charles and Diana equally, and especially Fergie, the former wife of Andrew. Their activities and outlandish public confessions irritated him. “My money is supporting that,” he would say. Nevertheless, Lincoln was a monarchist, waiting patiently for the next generation.

Lincoln invited me to his home on several occasions during the year. At a Christmas party in December, Karen Jurgens was at the door greeting the guests, and Lincoln was in the living room in his red bow tie and double-breasted blue coat. The trainees Peters and Ko, the anesthetists Scallan, Simpson, and Kehoe, and the pediatricians Shinebourne and Rigby, were there with or without spouses.

Originally from South Africa, Karen Jurgens was a tall, slender, very attractive brunette woman with a vivacious personality. She had a good sense of humor, and we shared many laughs together. I never inquired about her relationship with Lincoln, which was always strictly professional at work. Socially, she was at his side—the hostess of his parties, his companion on holidays abroad, and they seemed to enjoy each other's personality. They behaved so cordially and professionally toward one another at work that I did not discern their intimate relationship until she greeted me at his door at his Christmas party!

Melanie Cheung, Lincoln's secretary, and her soon-to-be fiancé Andrew Cohen were also there. Melanie was from Singapore, and Cohen was part English and part Spanish. He liked cigars and always offered one to me when we crossed paths. A cardiac surgery registrar at St. Mary's Hospital in London, Cohen trained briefly with Lincoln at the RBH, during which time he met Melanie, whom he subsequently invited on a date.

Also present was Dr. John Simons, a friend of Lincoln and the dentist of Lady Diana, of whom he said, "I don't know why Charles did not devote 18 hours a day to her. . . . She is always flirting with her eyes." Though not an oral surgeon by training, Simons surgically removed Diana's wisdom teeth. He felt aware of his professional colleagues watching the outcome of that operation. "In such a situation, everyone is waiting for you to fail," he told me. "You must identify your enemy." In a long conversation later over Stilton cheese and port, he said, "Don't believe your own myth. That is when the trouble comes." He had two sons: one an oral surgeon and one a dentist, and he was worried about them. "One is friendly on the outside and brittle on the inside, and one is brittle on the outside and weak on the inside."

One general practitioner was also there with his lovely wife from Switzerland. They regularly took holidays in France, he said, and yet he hated the French. Their son, Joshua Vecht, was a medical student spending a month in Los Angeles on the surgical team of Hillel Laks at UCLA. In January, Joshua came to work for Lincoln for a month. A polite and bright student, he gave us an informative talk on his experience at UCLA. After Lincoln asked him to prepare a talk for us, I urged Joshua to devote a considerable amount of time to it, knowing that this talk may be his best or only opportunity to speak before Lincoln. His observations of an American institution were interesting to hear. The chief resident in cardiothoracic surgery at UCLA at the time, Abbas Ardehali, was a classmate of mine at Emory University School of Medicine. I was pleased to hear that he had taken Joshua to a restaurant for lunch on his last day.

The food served at the Christmas party was impressive: suckling pig, roast beef with horseradish sauce, an open salmon, a plate of small cooked hens, new potatoes, tomatoes in an Italian dressing, and dishes of cranberry sauce and chutney. Champagne was served before dinner, red or white wine with dinner, and coffee and port after dinner. Lincoln emerged from the kitchen after dinner with a "Christmas pudding"—black plum pudding with cream sauce, aflame in brandy. When my turn came to be served, I asked, "What do you call this?" Lincoln stopped, stood up, and said to those near him, "Did you hear what he said?" Here was another opportunity to educate me.

His home at Pembroke Square was a four-story townhouse facing a central garden square, similar to those in Chelsea—and in Savannah, Georgia, for that matter. The kitchen and dining room were in the basement. One entered the front door to a hallway, and on the right was a formal living room with a fireplace. Coal- and wood-burning fires were outlawed in the homes of London because of pollution. A gas fire burned. The next floor up had an informal living room with a stereo system and bookshelves. I did not go beyond that floor. There were many clocks of all ages and shapes in both living rooms, and one heard the ticking of clocks in every room.

Lincoln showed me a painting of a boy about ten years old in the formal living room. This boy was his relative who died at 19 years of age while in the Aviation Corps during World War I. Sometime earlier, Lincoln had mentioned that he possessed some personal letters written by this young aviator, and he meant those letters when he said in front of the painting, "I will show you something else in a quieter moment."

Not long after arriving, I was speaking to a lady when Lincoln approached. "I am worried that this floor will fall out beneath you," he remarked, explaining that he had learned that day that the foundation was unstable. Another time I was talking with Dr. Simpson's wife with Lincoln when, after a few seconds of silence, he suddenly turned and walked away. Mrs. Simpson and I looked at one another quizically, but this was meant as no gesture of discourtesy. It was his usual manner.

My father visited in late December with Carrita Smith and her daughter, Ann Smith. Lincoln kindly invited us to his home at Pembroke Square for cocktails. He wore his usual bow tie, with a kerchief in his double-breasted blue jacket. Champagne was brought out on a silver tray, then a tray of slices of salmon rolled on toothpicks, and prawns in a biscuit cup. (By "biscuit" I do not mean cookie.) Karen Jurgens was also present in a lovely black dress, and Richard Sutton, a cardiologist with an expertise in pacemakers, was also there. Lincoln gave us a tour of his home (with the exception of the upstairs bedrooms) and the garden. The yard, which went back quite far, was green and dense and enclosed by brick walls on three sides. I had invited Lincoln to dine with us, but he persistently refused, not wishing to occupy the brief time of my visitors. My father left the next day, and Carrita Smith and I attended a delightful play called *An Inspector Calls,* by J. B. Priestly, at the Garrick Theater.

While living on Park Walk, I spent some time in the Dome Café on King's Road, around the corner from the Wilsons' home. It was a great place to read or write, with cappuccino and good music in the background. The days were cold in December, and my father bought me a tweed hat at James Lock and Co., "Hatters since 1676," at No. 6 St. James Street. While in this hat shop, I had my head "fitted" in a remarkable contraption that resembled a circular typewriter that would be gently placed on the head, the keys conforming to the cranium. The shape of my cranium was neither oval nor circular, but rather, asymmetric. I was told this was normal, and indeed, the cranial impressions of Oscar Wilde, Admiral Nelson, and others in the shop's display cabinet confirmed this. Next door on St. James Street was an old building with a plaque identifying the site of the "Texas Embassy," when the current state of Texas was the "Republic of Texas" from 1837 to 1844.

Chapter 12

Dr. Wilcox's Visit

My chief at Chapel Hill, Dr. Benson R. Wilcox, came in January to London, which had been his custom for over a decade. Staying at the Basil Street Hotel near Harrod's, he was joined by Mrs. Wilcox later in the week. Dr. Wilcox and Mr. Lincoln were about the same age, born in 1932 and 1933, respectively. Dr. Wilcox had lived all but four of his 64 years in North Carolina. He married Lucinda Holderness, another North Carolinian, in 1959, and they had four children who brought many grandchildren. After taking his college and medical education at UNC, Dr. Wilcox trained in surgery for seven years. He was then appointed Assistant Professor of Surgery in 1965 and full Professor six years later at age 39, the same age Mr. Lincoln became a Consultant.

Dr. Wilcox had been chief of the Division of Cardiothoracic Surgery at UNC for 27 years (since 1969) when I arrived to train in 1996. He had authored or co-authored some 170 articles and had confined his practice recently to pediatric cardiac surgery. His book with Professor Anderson, *Surgical Anatomy of the Heart,* was published in 1985 and was our guide at UNC in congenital heart disease. At his Friday morning conference, Dr. Wilcox regularly showed exquisite photographs of congenital cardiac malformations in children on whom he had operated during the previous week. His close professional collaboration with Professor Anderson obviously made it possible for me first to visit the Brompton in 1994 and then to work with Mr. Lincoln in 1996.

Dr. Wilcox and I shared an interest in history and books and maps. His medical history book collection, which he recently donated to the Health Sciences Library at UNC, was vast. In addition to the many books, his home in Chapel Hill had many old maps, several of North Carolina in particular, on the walls. Dr. Wilcox was always interested in the English language. One had to speak correctly. When I used the terms "basically" and "essentially" several times when presenting patients at one Friday morning conference, he instructed me immediately afterward to avoid the terms—"They're wasted words." One day I told him that I was "anxiously" awaiting a call from a pharmaceutical company. He said, "Do you mean 'eagerly'?" I looked forward to his visit in January to bring him up to date on my endeavors and tour London with him.

At the RBH he visited Professor Anderson, and then I gave him a tour of the ICUs and wards. He was impressed, as I was, by the particular attention given to patients by the nurses, and even suggested that we might arrange for one of our nurses at UNC to visit for a week and bring back ideas.

On Saturday, Dr. Wilcox invited me to join him at the Tate Gallery to hear a lecture by Laurence Bradbury, after which we took a taxi to the National Army Museum in Chelsea, which had fine exhibits on the World Wars. Then we went to Churchill's war rooms, which I had not seen. Walking past the Court of St. James, we made our way back to his lodgings.

Over sandwiches and tea at the Basil Street Hotel, he offered me a job at UNC, to begin upon my return to the States in August 1997. I was honored and elated. We discussed the probable salary range and what my role would be in the Division. It seemed ideal to me, and I accepted his offer. Before actually sitting down to tea, we had stopped by his room, where he retrieved a package. After our discussion, he gave me an old map of Georgia, "lest you should forget your roots."

During the next week, Dr. Wilcox frequented the operating theaters. He observed Lincoln performing a repair of tetralogy of Fallot in a 12-year-old boy, assisted by me. Fortunately, the operation went well. The next Saturday, Francis Ferdinand, the other American fellow, and I joined him at the Tate Gallery again for a lecture by Bradbury, followed by dinner that evening.

After Mrs. Wilcox joined him, I was invited to go with them to see *By Jeeves,* a comedy by Wodehouse, at the Lyric Theater. Wodehouse was one of Dr. Wilcox's favorite authors. We walked up the street after the play, and Mrs. Wilcox photographed my American mentor and me under a historic plaque of William Hunter, the great physician-scientist and brother of John Hunter, the so-called father of scientific surgery. The three of us then went to the Fountain Restaurant under Fortnum & Mason's and had a lively discussion over tea. Mrs. Wilcox reminded me of my mother's mother, Frances Carey Cansler of Charlotte, North Carolina, who spoke so engagingly of family. At one point, we discussed the effect of birth order on personality, stimulated by a new book on the subject called *Born to Rebel.*

Dr. Wilcox told me of his two experiences of living in England: the first in 1958 as a medical student working at Guy's Hospital, and the second in 1980 when he came with his family for an eight-month sabbatical to work with Professor Anderson at the RBH. At Guy's Hospital, he attended Brock's clinic and also observed, for the first time, a heart operation performed by Brock, with the assistance of Ross.

Dr. Wilcox said that he liked the British in general, but not always in the particular—which I took to mean that he liked many British institutions and traditions and manners, but not always the individual person. His heritage was Scotch-Irish and Presbyterian, many of whose kind settled in North and South Carolina. I mentioned that I was going to visit Dublin, and he recalled two incidents. During a city tour of Dublin, the guide proudly stated that Dublin kept its lights on at night during the bombing of Britain so that the Germans could use Dublin as a landmark on their way to bomb London. This offended the sensibilities of Wilcox. The other memory he shared was a tour of Trinity University, during which the guide repeatedly informed his audience that Trinity was "a Protestant university," not Catholic. Dr. Wilcox told me on the telephone later in the year that he toured the Guiness Brewery, where one is allowed to drink unlimited quantities of ale at the end of the tour.

As I mentioned earlier, Dr. Wilcox had developed a good working relationship with Professor Anderson, the cardiac morphologist at the RBH. Anderson had a gift for clarity and making sense of difficult concepts in congenital heart disease. In the weekly Monday morning meetings and in his courses, I learned a great deal from Anderson. In addition to his course in Liverpool in August, I took his two-day Foundation Course in Cardiac Morphology at the Conference Centre of the National Heart and Lung Institute in late February. Anderson was assisted by Drs. Gerlis, Ho, Smith, and Sheppard. The twenty or so attendees were separated into four tables, where we inspected the heart specimens.

Originally from Shropshire, Anderson was an avid golfer and an oenophile. His wife assisted him at work and, when he held video demonstrations in courses, she often managed the camera. He would speak of "this heart" or "this valuable specimen" as a fine example of tetralogy of Fallot or transposition of the great arteries. He disdained any alpha-numeric classifications of diseases. He never said "this is type I" or "type A" disease. Anderson presented the problem in plain English and advised one to "describe what you see." He also disdained Latin terminology, avoiding terms such as "sinus" or "conus" or "truncus arteriosus" or "ductus arteriosus" or "ligamentum arteriosum." He had an English term for each of the cardiac structures, normal or abnormal. Most of all, he did not like embryologic terms, such as "ostium primum" or "ostium secundum" defect. He associated embryologic terms with a rival cardiac morphologist from Harvard, van Praagh. During the year, Anderson encouraged me to write a paper on Tawara, a Japanese physician who studied the atrioventricular node during a two-year period in Germany. Tawara and his monograph on the conduction system of the heart have been little recognized except in Japan, but I was unable to bring myself to the task during the year.

Anderson had arrived at the Brompton in 1974, and soon thereafter, he and Lincoln studied the location of the sinus node in heart specimens. Anderson told me that Lincoln had "no arrhythmia complications" after the Mustard operation (atrial switch operation for transposition of the great arteries), of which he did many. Lincoln used to say that Anderson was a "luxury" at the RBH. Toward the end of my year, he noticed that Anderson was more disputatious than usual in Monday morning conference. "Charles, I am worried about him," Lincoln would say. "Something is wrong." We speculated that his professional relationship with The University of Pittsburgh had ended recently and he was disturbed that he would no longer be taking yearly sabbaticals abroad.

Chapter 13

St. Luke's Street

In late January, I left for my second trip home, arriving in Chapel Hill on Thursday, January 30. Lydia and I dined together, delighted to see one another. The next day, I gave a talk on the modified Blalock-Taussig shunt to the The Nathan A. Womack Surgical Society of UNC, which was holding its biennial meeting in Chapel Hill. Lydia and I attended a black tie dinner by the Womack Society that night, and I spent most of the next several days studying for my written board examinations in thoracic surgery.

On Wednesday, February 5, I went to Nashville and spent two days with my daughters, Amelia and Camille. Camille was sick on Thursday, and so the two of us spent the day together at the library while Amelia attended school. Cliff Roberts, my older brother, arrived Thursday night, and we all dined on fried chicken and mashed potatoes and gravy at the Loveless Restaurant outside of Nashville. The following day we drove to Georgia, stopping on the way at Lookout Mountain, the Civil War battlefield near Chattanooga. We also stopped briefly at the Holbrook Campground and Cemetery in North Georgia, which had been established by our ancestors.

The following day, I reluctantly parted from Amelia and Camille and Cliff's family and went to the Hilton Hotel at the Atlanta airport. On Sunday morning, I took Part I of the American Board of Thoracic Surgery Examination, which was long and grueling. This drudgery was balanced, however, by the pleasure of seeing Jim Zellner, my old friend from general surgery days at the Medical University of South Carolina at Charleston, and Patrick Griffith, the cardiothoracic fellow who preceded me at Chapel Hill and whose lovely wife Petronilla had introduced me to

Lydia. On Sunday night, February 9, I returned to London, arriving on Monday morning.

Because of Lydia's impending move to London, I vacated Neville Street and took a one-bedroom flat for six months at 21 St. Luke's Street, which ran parallel to Sydney Street, behind St. Luke's Church. Just one block from the RBH (even closer than Neville Street), it was an ideal location. I paid about £950 per month ($1600) to live there, but by taking call at the hospital every fourth night, I tripled my salary. Although my financial status was not good, it was not desperate.

The flat at 21 St. Luke's Street was in the basement of a townhouse owned by Charles and Errol Elizabeth Slee. The flat had a small living room, a small bedroom with a double bed, a kitchen, and a bathroom. A back door entered upon a private garden, which looked out on the public garden adjacent to St. Luke's Church. The entrance to the flat was rather uninviting, as one had to walk downstairs and lower one's head to get in the door, as I painfully learned. These several months on St. Luke's Street were perhaps my happiest period, especially after Lydia arrived.

Errol Slee communicated by notes occasionally to notify me when she and her husband were leaving town. I entered their rooms through a communicating door to retrieve my mail, "to check my post," when they were away. Errol's notes kept me abreast of the household activities: "Roy, our longstanding builder, will be in our house decorating our bedroom." Lincoln used to say that I was very lucky to find the flat on St. Luke's Street with its proximity to the RBH.

In the asphalt-covered park to the right of St. Luke's Church, there were soccer games in the evening, which I enjoyed watching. The Olympics in Atlanta had just concluded when I arrived in London in August, and the athleticism of the British was a subject of concern. Known for their love of "sport," the British had fared miserably in the recent Olympics, and several government officials expressed the intent to reorganize the Olympic training programs in particular, and school-level athletics in general.

Lincoln was in good shape physically for his age—he was slim and strong, with a good deal of physical endurance. He said often that cardiac surgery is very physically demanding. The British people in general, however, were not natural athletes, at least the ones I watched playing soccer beside St. Luke's Church. They had pluck and perseverance and they loved the game, but natural athletes were "as rare as hen's teeth," as Professor Anderson would say. If basketball players were taken randomly off the high school playground in the States and compared with those off the soccer fields in the UK, the Americans may have a slight edge. But this is changing, of course, as the American teenager stays indoors with the computer and television and becomes obese. I do not doubt, however, the mental toughness of the English.

On the opposite side of St. Luke's Church was a green garden park that backed up to our flat. At one end of St. Luke's Street was the Builders Pub, and at the other end on the corner was the Blenheim Pub, which was more appealing to Lydia and me. Many Sundays during the year, I attended the service at St. Luke's Church. The Reverend Derek Watson was engaging, but he left the parish in the fall. Various ministers substituted until a permanent replacement was found. A minister one Sunday spoke on being sensitive to the suffering in the world, and he began his sermon with the eloquent words, "May I speak in the name of the Father, Son, and Holy Ghost," then crossed himself. The number of parishioners at church at 11 a.m. was small, which was consistent with the trend of Anglicans not attending church in the UK. I read in *The Times* that the UK will have more mosque-going Muslims than church-going Christians in 20 years.

I was not exposed to evangelical Christianity at St. Luke's Church on Sydney Street. The sermons were thoughtful and intelligent in general, and, of course, the beautiful *Book of Common Prayer* dominated the service. I was intrigued by the memorials to British soldiers from the parish. Every cushion that one knelt upon to pray had the embroidered name of a fallen British soldier. Regimental flags from various wars were framed upon the walls of the chapel. I had not seen this in the States. One sees statues and war memorials in the town square, but not in the church.

During her four months in London, Lydia had two jobs. One was at a specialty toy store on Cale Street, where she worked about twice a week for several hours each time. The owner would often leave her alone in the store with a key. Although the job was not terribly exciting, it afforded Lydia an opportunity to meet English people coming in to shop. The store was only two blocks from our flat, which was very convenient.

Her other job was with Lorraine Spencer, who employed her to care for her three children at their home in Notting Hill. Lorraine was married to a wealthy businessman who traveled frequently, and Lydia spent a good deal of time at their home. Coincidentally, Karen Jurgens, the surgical assistant, was good friends with Lorraine Spencer's former nanny. The oldest boy was away at boarding school much of the time, so Lydia usually took care of the second boy, Thomas, and his little sister, Alexandra. She often picked them up from school, fixed them dinner, bathed them, and put them to bed. She and Lorraine became good friends, and Lorraine kindly attended our small wedding ceremony in July.

Leslie Jeng, Francis Ferdinand's fiancée, and Lydia spent many hours together. Both were interested in paintings, and they often went to the Tate and National Galleries. Leslie had already been living in London for a while and took Lydia to all her favorite places. In April they met in Berlin for a weekend, the first time Lydia had visited the Continent. Lydia was impressed with the extent of reconstruction in East Berlin, remarking when she had looked up in the sky, dozens of cranes appeared. On another weekend, Lydia and Leslie went to Scotland on a bus tour. They returned with harrowing tales of the journey because the bus was much smaller than they expected and the tour guide had never been to Scotland! Sharon Aldridge, a friend of Lydia's from Wilmington, North Carolina, came to visit Lydia for a week in June, and they visited Paris together. In all, Lydia saw Prague, Berlin, Edinburgh, Paris, and Nice, as well as Birmingham, Bath, and Cambridge, not bad for a four-month stay in London!

Chapter 14

Views of America

Views of the USA held by Europeans that I heard during the year ranged widely. Most Europeans I worked with tended to view the States unfavorably and expressed criticism occasionally if an opportunity arose. From those Europeans who had actually lived in the States for a significant period of time, however, I rarely heard sharp criticism or naive generalizations. The barrage of minor and occasionally major insults usually came from those who had significant gaps in their knowledge of America. They had only visited—perhaps for two weeks in Florida or one week at a medical meeting in California or to see a relative for a week in Boston, etc. Similarly, an American who had spent a week in East London, or perhaps a week at the Lake District, or a week in a hotel in Birmingham for a medical meeting would be unqualified to generalize about daily life in England.

The greatest European misunderstanding of the USA was that Americans were alike all over the country, i.e., that there is a homogenized American who holds certain distinct views (presented to Europeans by Hollywood). Few seemed aware of the widely diverse backgrounds of Americans—that African-Americans comprise 12% of the population, Hispanic-Americans 11%, and Asian-Americans 5%, and that these percentages vary widely depending on whether one lives in rural Vermont or San Diego or Charleston, South Carolina. The proportion of Americans not of European descent is approaching half. One friend, upon returning from San Francisco, remarked to me that she saw many Oriental people, but that she didn't see many "Americans." I reminded her that those Oriental people *were* Americans.

The second knowledge gap of non-Americans was an understanding of the immense size of the USA, such that life in a little town in

Georgia may be quite different from life in south central Los Angeles, or on a farm in Kansas, or in a working class blue-collar neighborhood in Pittsburgh. The state of Georgia is the size of England and Wales combined, and Texas is the size of France. Innumerable times I heard someone say, "They do this in America"—often referring to something I had never done or even seen done.

Lincoln, who had lived in the States for a year, never once insulted the USA in my presence, which distinguished him among those I worked with. I think Lincoln grasped precisely those two points about the States: that its people are diverse and that the landscape is immense. But of course Lincoln drove across the country and saw it for himself in 1968.

He remarked once on an article on the USA in the Saturday edition of the *Financial Times*. The reporter suggested that Americans should be more proud of their heritage than they appear to be, particularly when dealing with other countries. One example cited in the article was how Clinton, with his broken leg, was taken down from the airplane in a *catering truck,* rather than in a more dignified way. In his interaction with Yeltsin during their meeting in Finland during the spring of 1997, Clinton could have very easily assumed the moral high ground, according to Lincoln. Russia is nearly twice as large in land area as the USA, and yet the productivity in the USA far outweighs the productivity of Russia. Lincoln believed "it is because of hard work."

Apart from an occasional vacation in the States, the chief method of acquiring information on the USA by most people in the UK appeared to be from television or Hollywood movies. For example, "ER"—a show about fictitious characters in a fictitious emergency room of an indigent care hospital in Chicago—had a large British audience, and yet I knew few people at home who watched it. An endless stream of Hollywood movies appeared in the cinemas (theaters) in Chelsea. Many non-Americans seem to forget, however, that most Americans go to work, raise families, travel little on their two weeks of vacation a year, and do not experience the extraordinary events that form the basis of so many Hollywood movies.

Many people took little thought about criticizing America in the presence of an American. For example, Francis Ferdinand, my American friend, once said at the table, "I want to go to the Lake District before summer, when so many American tourists come." The Australian nurse said immediately, "Oh God, awful!" in the presence of two Americans, as if we were not to be offended. And yet I don't think Ferdinand would have made a cutting remark about Australian tourists in the presence of two Australians. At a pub once I commented on the many different countries from which our group haled. A cardiology nurse remarked, "Yes, she's from Finland, he's from Cyprus, he's from Pakistan, she's from Canada, and he's from God-knows-where," knowing I was from the States. It was a strangely accepted practice among the less educated to criticize the USA openly in the presence of an American.

A humorous episode that occurred early one evening in the operating theater lounge illustrates the paradoxical view of Europeans toward the States. "Beavis and Butthead," the MTV (Music Television) American cartoon comedy, was showing on television when I walked in, and I attempted to change it to the news. An Irish perfusionist was glued to the cartoon and insisted that we keep it on "Beavis and Butthead." Moments later, an Irish senior registrar appeared and sat down and criticized us for watching this "American culture," unaware that his own countryman had insisted on watching it!

I encountered no one during my entire year in London with whom I could hold a dialogue on American history. This experience supports a passage I read in a book by Stefan Potter called *Potter on America* (1956). This Englishman wrote that "mutual disapproval is due to mutual ignorance. Knowledge of the history of the United States, most rewarding of subjects, is the intelligent Englishman's biggest gap." No one with whom I interacted on a regular basis had much knowledge of the three or four essential events in American history. I don't mean to suggest that I *expected* anyone to have this knowledge, but it does confirm the observation of Stefan Potter. Certainly, the same observation could be made by Europeans about most Americans' lack of knowledge of European history, let alone Asian or African history. Many of my countrymen do not know their own history!

Hollywood movies and television have projected upon the typical European a picture of the USA that is both light and superficial, lacking in manners and traditions. Europeans tended to view their own lives as deeper and heavier, steeped in traditions and manners. And yet I found this view often at odds with reality. Most of my American friends of 20 years or more appear to me to be more steeped in traditions and manners than their European counterparts of the same generation. But perhaps the traditions and manners were there; I simply did not recognize them.

Many Europeans had a skewed view of the sensibilities of the average American. One German surgeon who had never been to the States told me at a pub with all seriousness that "divorce is nothing to an American" because the divorce rate in the States is now about 40 per cent. I was reminded of Stalin's famous comment, "One death is a tragedy; one million is a statistic," which could be applied to divorce. Perhaps the German's view was derived from Hollywood, where multiple divorces are more common and the consequences appear insignificant to a European across the ocean.

Lincoln spoke often of his research year at the Massachusetts General Hospital in Boston in 1968. He was most grateful for the experience and the hospitality he received. Several times Lincoln said to me about my year in London, "Charles, this will be the greatest year of your life," and perhaps he was also saying this about his own year abroad. He worked in the experimental laboratory of Dr. Gerald Austen, primarily on lung research. Shortly after furnishing and settling into an apartment in Boston, he found he had spent his life savings. He went to see Austen, the chairman of surgery, who said to him, "I know why you're here. You need money," and Austen immediately helped him.

Mortimer Buckley, another cardiac surgeon at Massachusetts General Hospital at the time, was, according to Lincoln, the first Irish-Catholic chief resident in surgery at the "Mass General." He had been educated at Boston University, not Harvard. During our conversation on my first day in his office, Lincoln said, "I think Mortimer Buckley held me personally responsible for the British occupation of Northern Ireland. I represented to him the evil face of British Imperialism."

Lincoln related one amusing episode in the Harvard laboratory. He had just anesthetized a dog, which then suddenly began to vomit. Not wanting the dog to aspirate vomitus into its lungs, Lincoln picked up the dog by its hind legs and held it upside down. Just as vomitus was spilling onto Lincoln's clothes, Austen and a prominent trustee of the Massachusetts General Hospital appeared at the door, and Austen kindly introduced the trustee to Lincoln, "our visiting surgeon from England."

The last five weeks of his year in the States, Lincoln bought an old car and drove it to California. He remembered sleeping in the car one night in one of the western states. Awakened by a state trooper, Lincoln said, "I lifted my eyelids and was staring at a revolver through the window." The trooper told him that it was illegal to sleep in his car there and that a motel was "just down the road." Lincoln remarked, "'Just down the road,' of course, meant 100 miles." Lincoln recalled that the license plates in certain western states have phrases like "Big Sky Country," and he said, "It is true. The skylines and the sunsets I observed in the West were amazing." Lincoln also said, "Even at the end of my year in Boston, I did not fully comprehend the size and distance across America—just how large the country is."

But the British were "spot on" (from "spot on the dot" which means, on target) about some aspects of American life. Tony Desouza teased constantly about the obesity in the States—all the fat Americans! I did not fully appreciate his observation until I opened my eyes to it on visits home. Europeans clearly stay closer to ideal body weight, for whatever reason. Europeans smoke more, but the fact is that they eat less. A third of Americans are obese by recent American criteria; by international criteria, over half of Americans are obese. Lincoln recalled that during his year of research in Boston, he would go to the coffee shop at the Massachusetts General Hospital at about 3 p.m. "to get away from the smell of the lab. I would watch people eat blueberry pie," he said, "as if it was their last meal on earth." I asked him if he ate only one meal a day at that time, and he responded affirmatively.

The British tended to be more quiet and private than Americans. Not infrequently, the American will tell you what he or she thinks, whether you care to know it or not. The American will ask you personal questions unabashedly or will be aggressively friendly, sometimes to the point of irritation. The American may know very little about the world and yet will issue bold opinions, confident that they are worth hearing. Environments inhabited by Americans tend to be louder. This was true inside and outside of the operating room.

The British, in my experience of one year, tended to work quietly and efficiently. They were not outspoken with their views and tended to respect one another's privacy. This cultural difference came about, in part, I believe, because Great Britain is a small island which is densely populated. Its people must behave in a civilized way or chaos will reign. The USA, in contrast, is less densely populated. England fits into North Carolina, and the population of London (7 million) is roughly the same as that spread out over the state of North Carolina, the 10th most populated of the 50 states. It has not been "necessary" for Americans to be courteous and reserved. Americans like to bring attention to themselves.

The British I met knew more about the world, in general, than most Americans I knew. But this had much to do with the British Empire, which introduced into English life aspects of different cultures in the world. The English still view the world as their oyster, in some ways.

When visiting the Victoria and Albert Museum, Lydia and I were guided by an Englishman of about 60 years of age. He conveyed a good deal of information to us during the tour. In a great hall, he showed us an enormous cast of the Roman Emperor Trajan's column. He said that the British had to make plaster casts of the entire original column in Italy, and the process was incredibly laborious, involving high scaffolds around the tall column. It sounded like an extraordinary feat of art and engineering, and I was somewhat surprised that the Italians permitted such a time-consuming spectacle at one of their artistic treasures. I asked the English guide how the British were allowed to do this in Italy. He looked at me quizically and said, “There was no other way.” In other words, there was no other way to make the replica than to build the scaffolds around the column and pour the plaster. That Italians might object was not even a consideration.

But the differences in temperament and attitude are slowly diminishing, I suspect, under the leveling influence of the television and computer, which has begun to unify and homogenize the world. Certainly a man of Lincoln’s manners and habits, formed before the television and computer age, belongs to England. The younger generation was less distinctively English, just as the next generation of Americans may be more worldly.

Chapter 15

English Cuisine

About once a week, I craved an English breakfast—baked beans, steamed mushrooms, a cooked tomato, a length of sausage and a slice of ham, with two fried eggs, all served with toast with butter and jelly, and coffee. On several occasions, I was encouraged to try the "black pudding," which was blood formed into a sausage, but declined at each opportunity. In Dublin I was once served "white pudding," which was plasma formed into a sausage. It was tasty, but I only tasted. Cyrus Wilson, my American friend, developed the same taste for the English breakfast, which he enjoyed every Sunday at the Dome Cafe on King's Road.

I ate more "chips" (French fries) during the year than the cumulative total in my entire life. Chips were served in the cafeteria at every meal, and it was the typical accompanying vegetable to the entree, whether it was mince-meat pie, shepherd's pie, lamb, or chicken. A typical dinner was sausage with grilled onions, baked beans, and chips. Another was lamb with green mint jelly with chips. One had to grasp quickly that "chips" were French fries, "crisps" were potato chips, and "biscuits" were cookies. I still do not know what American-type biscuits are called in England! It helped to know that "sultana" were raisins and "aubergine" was eggplant. "Starter" was used in the UK for appetizer, and the British often used the word "meal," which is rarely used in the States. Let's go out for a "meal" would be said, instead of let's go out for lunch or dinner.

The influence of Indian cuisine in London was obvious. Curry-flavored dishes were served in the cafeteria on a regular basis. I usually had the chicken curry over rice, which was routinely better than the beef. I also liked saag, a Hindu dish of potatoes and spinach. Tandoori chicken and coronation chicken were also served occasionally.

Cheese and crackers usually followed, rather than preceded, dinner, and Stilton cheese with port was an after-dinner tradition on special occasions. Waitrose, the grocery store, had a variety of English cheeses, such as Leicester and Cheshire, which were new to my palate. I loved clotted cream from Cornwall, though it is bad for the arteries. Cornish pastry often accompanied it. One of my few regrets was not visiting Cornwall, the southwesternmost shire of England, the family seat of Lord Cornwallis, the British general who failed to subdue the Carolinas in the Revolutionary War.

The variety of sandwiches offered in the cafeterias and in the stores was amazing. One could buy chicken tandoori and cucumber, chicken mayonnaise and sweet corn, etc. I ate a good deal of lamb during the year, whereas I probably ate lamb only once a year in the USA. I remember remarking to Lincoln that lamb was the sort of thing one ate at the Sir Walter Raleigh Inn in Williamsburg at Thanksgiving, not at the usual evening meal.

Just before I arrived in London, several persons became infected with a deadly virus after eating British beef. Continental Europeans suddenly protested the importation of British beef, and farmers everywhere were in an uproar, which finally settled down—it had no impact on my culinary experience. Restaurants would often advertise in the window that they did or did not serve British beef. It seemed to be a mark of patriotism to serve it.

Needless to say, I drank large quantities of tea during the year and became somewhat familiar with the various types—English Breakfast, Earl Grey, Darjeeling, Ceylon, etc. Thomas Twining opened his tea shop in London in 1717, and I bought Twining's tea at Waitrose during the year. Francis Ferdinand told me several times that he bought his tea at Harrod's. Surprisingly, it was reported that the British now drink more coffee than tea. I partook of the British tea ceremony in late afternoon a few times during the year, specifically at Brown's Hotel in Mayfair, The Pelham Hotel in South Kensington, and the Fountain Restaurant at the Fortnum and Mason store. Lydia, my fiancée, told me that Lorraine Spencer, for whom she worked, would regularly call her children to "tea" in the evening, which was "supper" in the States, a term I never heard in the UK.

Champagne was often enjoyed before dinner, whereas I rarely drank it at home. I never saw anyone drink bourbon, and only rarely did someone order Scotch. Whiskey seemed to be served much more in the States. I never enjoyed the dark beers, finding the Guiness in Dublin too heavy, usually restricting myself to half a pint of beer (one glass) at a pub. It was common practice to offer to buy others a drink when you went to get one for yourself. The pubs were gathering points, and on a weekly basis we met after work at the Wellesley Arms Pub, across the street from the RBH. Melanie Cheung, Lincoln's secretary, often would arrange it. Everyone would usually meet around 6 p.m. and leave within a couple of hours.

David Jones, the cardiothoracic resident at UNC two years after me, once remarked that he couldn't stand the English pubs because of the smoke. I took this into consideration during my year in London; the air was indeed heavy with smoke, but it did not generally bother me. The Europeans I interacted with smoked cigarettes much more frequently than my American friends at home.

Lincoln routinely requested that I buy him Gauloise unfiltered cigarettes at Heathrow on my travels. With every good intention of buying him his particular brand of cigarettes, I failed every time—the duty-free store had just run out of them, or they never carried them, or I forgot to buy them in Heathrow *before* departing and could not re-enter the duty-free stores upon returning. I always had some excuse, and Lincoln jokingly remarked that a moral objection kept me from buying them. Of course Lincoln believed one should be allowed to pursue one's vices, *any* vices, after 60 years of age.

The operating theater routinely provided dinner for the on-call surgical registrar, as well as anyone in the operating theater working past 7:00 p.m. The styrofoam dinner containers usually contained meat pies with chips, or sausage and chips and beans, or tandoori chicken with rice. Occasionally, a hamburger with chips appeared, or a sort of vegetable salad. For dessert, there was always sponge cake with custard. Custard was poured over all desserts, usually enhancing an otherwise dull cake.

In general, restaurant service in London was not as attentive as it was at home. In the States, one became accustomed to waiters and waitresses eager to please, whereas the attitude in London was more indifferent. The posture in London seemed to be, "It is a privilege for you to eat in our restaurant," whereas at home the attitude was more often, "It is a privilege for us to serve you in our restaurant." I remarked on this to Tony Desouza, and he confirmed the observation, adding that Londoners are too polite and need to be more demanding at restaurants. The best service Lydia and I experienced was with Tony and Sarah Desouza at Stepping Stone, a restaurant in Queen's Town serving modern British cuisine.

Strange comments on American food were frequent. Once again, they were usually made by persons who had never lived in the States. I stood before the hospital cafeteria cashier one day at noon with a bowl of cereal for "lunch"—something I had never done before. The Malaysian cashier said to me, "Oh, that's typical American, to eat cereal for lunch." In fact, I cannot ever remember seeing anyone eat cereal for lunch in 36 years! Most Europeans concluded after their vacation in Florida that "Americans eat an enormous breakfast"—true for many people, and yet the English breakfast of two fried eggs, baked beans, mushrooms, sausage and ham, plus toast struck me as huge.

I once commented to a group of nurses who were eating at the nurses station that what they call "bacon," we would call ham—that our "bacon" was cut into thin strips and fried until it was brown and crispy. An Irish nurse did not hesitate to point out that that was because "Americans don't know how to cook." Many times I was tempted to point out to my English or Irish friends that there were virtually no "English" or "Irish" restaurants in the States, whereas there were many American restaurants in London. One had only to walk down King's Road to find an American "diner," or a New Orleans-style restaurant serving Cajun food, or the usual McDonald's, which was always crowded, or a Texas-style barbecue restaurant up the street. And yet most Europeans think Americans eat hamburgers and French fries every night. One friend said to me, "There are no Indian restaurants in America, are there?", to which I replied, "There are four on Franklin Street in Chapel Hill, North Carolina," not to mention the restaurants serving Italian, Greek, Chinese, and Mexican food.

On Old Brompton Road were two Indian restaurants side by side: Nizam and the Star of India. The Wilsons took me to Nizam in late August, a month after I arrived in London. It was my first and best Indian culinary experience. Though the Indian appetizers were unappealing to me, the bread and the main courses were delicious. I had lamb with a cream sauce called Korma, over rice. I went there with my mother, Bob, and Frances later in the year. The Star of India was slightly larger and more expensive. When my father visited in October, we went there with Luke Glancy the first night.

The Bombay Brasserie near the Gloucester Road tube station was the third fine Indian restaurant I enjoyed. As I mentioned earlier, Luke Glancy took his cardiology associates there as a farewell gesture, and he invited me. When my father came in May, we hosted a dinner for Lincoln there, as well. Lincoln pointed out to me the large framed photographs of the British in India during the Empire years. It was a time of opulence and ceremony, which these photographs captured.

I went to numerous other restaurants with the Wilsons during the year. In August, we dined together at La Famiglia on Langeton Street in Chelsea, a short walk from their home. We ate there together twice more during the year, and the Italian owners knew the Wilsons. I ate wild boar for the first time. Lydia and I also had a delightful Italian dinner with the Wilsons at the Sambuca Restaurant on Symond Street near Cadogon Square. It was the first time Lydia had met the Wilsons.

Twice I had fish at Live Bait, opposite the Young Vic. The first time was with Luke Glancy and his son Mark, after seeing *Long Day's Journey Into Night.* We devoured plates of prawns, which are smaller than the shrimp off the American coast. I had broiled cod and potatoes. Of course, Dr. Glancy was from New Orleans and appreciated good food. The star actress of the play dined a few tables over from us. I returned to Live Bait with my father and Lydia. After walking halfway across London, we lunched at Live Bait with white wine, then walked down the street to the Old Vic and saw Oscar Wilde's *An Ideal Husband,* a splendid choice, as my father and I were soon to be married. The wine had its effect upon us, as we each dozed off at times during the play. After that experience, I made it a point to rest during the day and eat lightly before a play.

Several times I had Thai food at the Bangkok Restaurant off Old Brompton Road when visitors came. Toward the end of the year, Francis Ferdinand and I dined at S & P Thai Restaurant on Fulham Road. Francis was always a pleasure to dine with because he knew something about food and wine, his conversation was usually lively, and he certainly relished the cuisine.

One obvious difference in dining technique between the British and Americans was how the utensils are held. The British hold the fork in the left hand and the knife in the right. Food is swept onto the fork or smeared onto the fork, depending on the food, and then the fork is brought to the mouth, still in the left hand. Surprisingly, the fork is often upside down as it rises to the mouth, with food positioned on its backside. The whole process struck me as odd, and even coarse, but I tried it now and then experimentally, with good effect. One of the consequences of such a two-handed technique is that the clatter of cutlery rings throughout the room. It is not typically quiet dining at an English table. Even little elderly ladies generate a racket feeding themselves. Asians from the former British colonies also ate with this technique.

In contrast, I was bred to raise the fork to my mouth with the right hand. I may prepare the steak morsels with fork in left and knife in right, but always the food was presented to my mouth on the fork in its upright position in the right hand. How this difference in technique evolved in the two countries I do not know. Perhaps Americans began to hold bread in their left hand during dinner, as my grandfather evidently did, forcing the fork to the right.

To dine on true dinner plates and silverware in the RBH cafeteria was a relief. The cafeteria at UNC Hospitals had gone to styrofoam plates and plastic utensils before I left because the silverware was getting stolen. The British were also adamant about having a saucer with their teacup. The teacups, saucers, and spoons rattled away in conference.

Chapter 16

The London Language

Within a few days of arriving in London, I attended a "barbeque party" hosted by the RBH. Having made no friends yet, I appeared at this party on the patio of the hospital dormitory, in which many doctors and nurses and others lived who worked at the RBH. To my surprise, I saw no physicians the entire night, soon realizing that this party was intended for the various staff of the hospital—the cooks in the cafeteria, porters, technicians, etc. Nevertheless, I engaged in conversation a 25-year-old poor woman from a nearby housing project, called Council Housing in the UK. She was a friend of a friend of a friend of an employee at the hospital. She took illicit drugs regularly, had no job, and was on welfare. Her two sons were being raised by her mother somewhere in Chelsea. What amazed me was that I comprehended only a third of her speech, which was peppered with Cockney expressions. Though we both lived in English-speaking countries, her speech was foreign to me. This was a dramatic and severe introduction to the English language in London.

Most Londoners spoke faster than I was accustomed to, but the voice was usually clear and the vocabulary, in general, better than in the States. Several expressions were routinely used in daily conversation. "Oh, right!" was a sort of response, as in: "I'm hungry." "Oh, right!" Or: "A train crashed in Manchester." "Oh, right!" Or: "We need to operate on that patient now." "Oh, right!" It was an acknowledging statement, just as the words "all right" were often used as a greeting. A fellow surgeon who saw me in the morning would say, "All right, Charles?" "Yes," I would say, "I'm all right, thank you."

One heard the word "bit" in conversation regularly. "We've done our bit." A note to me from the maid on Park Walk read: "Happy New

Year. Don't forget bits on table." By "bits" she meant the socks and underwear. An echocardiogram would be shown at Monday morning conference, and Shinebourne would remark, "Show us that bit in the right hand corner again, Manjit." I think Americans use thing in place of "bit." The word "proper" was commonly used. "He'll work at the Brompton until he can find a proper job" or "We can't do that procedure at the bedside, she needs a proper operation."

Lincoln was fond of saying "just there—place the stitch just there." Or, looking at a map, "I'm going just there." Karen Jurgens pointed out to me that people also say "just now"—"I will be there just now." Lincoln often said, "Don't worry," by which he meant "I don't want to hear any more." He would often say it to nurses who were telling him about a problem or to someone expressing concern about the schedule. Lincoln would also say, "That's it." When he had just put in the last stitch: "That's it." Or, if a situation appeared futile: "That's it. I can do no more."

Certain expressions one heard regularly around the hospital, such as "organize it." The senior registrar would turn to the nurse and say, "Why don't you organize that x-ray and I'll come back in 30 minutes to review it?" Or a nurse would say, "I am going to organize a party in two weeks." The word "happy" was used a lot. The registrar would look at the patient and then the nurse and say to her, "Are you happy?" She would say enthusiastically, "Yes, he'll go home today." Lincoln never said "Are you happy?" But a nurse might look at me as I was looking over a patient and say, "Happy?" One says Happy Christmas in London, not Merry Christmas.

The nurses often described patients as "settled," meaning calm and stable, or "unsettled," particularly when describing a child. The terms "well" and "unwell" were also used frequently, whereas one rarely heard them in the States. "Review" the patient meant to evaluate the patient, another term never heard in that context in the States. "Nil by mouth" of course meant nothing by mouth. A child was "cyanosed" (blue), not cyanotic. A patient was "breathless," not short of breath.

Several medical terms caught me off guard. "Tubes" was used interchangeably with stethoscope. A "bleeper" was a beeper. A "drain" was a chest tube. "Pipes" were cannulas. "Sash" was used by Lincoln for tubing. "Divide the sash," he would say at operation. Some surgical instruments had different names. A "newt" was a peanut in the States. A "clip" was a tag or mosquito. "Touch forceps." as Lincoln called them, were DeBakey forceps. An "eyelid retractor" was a vein retractor, a "nerve hook" was an eyelid retractor, and a "Blalock hook," as Lincoln called it, was a nerve hook in the States.

Of course a surgeon was addressed as "Mister," not doctor, and he had his "list," meaning his operating schedule. Melanie might call and say, "Charles, a patient for mitral valve replacement has been added to Mr. Lincoln's list tomorrow." Lincoln saw his private patients in "his rooms" on Harley Street. The medical record of each patient was called the patient's "notes." A "chest physician" was a pulmonologist, and a "chest infection" was pneumonia. The nurse would say the child's chest sounds "grotty," meaning unclear, or she might say he sounds "chesty," which may be a little better, but still abnormal. When the supplemental oxygen was discontinued, the patient was "breathing air," whereas an American would say, he is on room air.

The nurse might say "I have bled him," and she didn't mean therapeutic bleeding as was practiced 200 years ago. She meant "I have drawn blood from one of his veins for tests." She might also say that the patient's bowels have not "opened," while an American would say moved.

The cardiologist would say the patient had an "ejection systolic murmur," not a systolic ejection murmur. It was heard at the left sternal "edge," not border, as in the States. "Adrenaline" was epinephrine, and "noradrenaline" was norepinephrine. Coronary arteries were not occluded, they were "blocked." The surgeon sewed the "bottom ends," meaning distal anastomoses, then the "top ends," meaning proximal anastomoses. The nurse circulator in the operating theater was called the "runner." The porter went to "collect" the patient. I suppose the orderly went to get the patient in the States.

The phrase "having said that" was also commonly heard in conference: "I think the patient has terrible ventricular function, and his outlook, even with an operation, is dismal. Having said that, I think Mr. Lincoln should operate on the child tomorrow." "Together with" is another expression regularly said on the eastern side of the Atlantic. "The cardiac surgeons, together with the cardiologists, have recommended an operation."

"Hmm" was frequently used in place of "yes." All Englishmen use the expression, some with greater frequency than others. As I mentioned earlier, Jeremy Prout, the senior house officer from Somerset, used the expression regularly, yet Lincoln rarely used it. Lincoln often said, "As you say," which was commonly heard at conferences. I liked the expression, because it acknowledged that one heard what the other person said and confirmed it. Lincoln might say in conference, "As you say, his prognosis is dismal, but I shall operate to relieve his symptoms."

Lincoln, like other Englishmen, would also use the word "pity," which is rarely used in the States. "It's a pity, really," he would say, or

"What a pity." Tony Desouza and others would often use the expression "meant to be." The patient was "meant to be operated on yesterday, but he never appeared at hospital." The expressions "should do" or "could do" were also used. "Shall we operate on Mr. Smith tomorrow? . . . Could do." "Will Mr. Lincoln be doing that arterial switch on Friday? . . . Should do." Paul Peters always used "whilst" for while. An Englishman would not make a long story short, he would "cut" it short. Lincoln would "touch wood" for luck, whereas Americans knock on wood.

The word "sorry" is repeated throughout the day by people from all walks of life. "Sorry" can mean, "Excuse me for bumping into you," or it can be posed as a question to mean "I didn't hear you. Please repeat what you said." A senior registrar mumbles to the nurse, "Pull out his chest drains this morning." Not hearing him, she responds, "Sorry?" and so he repeats it louder. I have also heard "sorry" used as a kind of apology for interrupting or trying to make a point. Shinebourne might become agitated in Monday morning conference during a heated discussion and say, "Sorry. Sorry. I'm so sorry. This child is terribly unwell and, I think, needs surgical repair." I found "sorry" irritating at first, but grew accustomed to its frequent use as another example of the politeness of British society.

"I would have thought" is another common expression I never heard at home. "I would have thought the weather would clear by now." "I would have thought the Germans would attack by now." Lincoln was often saying "Oh no, no, no, no, no" or "Oh yes, yes, yes, yes, yes." I heard the expression "Thanks very much indeed" on a regular basis. One would see a patient and tell him that he must stay in the hospital at least another week, and he would respond, "Thanks very much indeed." The little old English lady would be instructed by the postman to place a 63 pence stamp on the envelope, and she would respond, "With pleasure. . . . Thanks very much indeed."

The phrase "sort it out" startled my sensibilities more than any other expression. It was used in a variety of ways. A senior registrar would say "I have to go up and sort out Mr. Jones on Alexander Ward," meaning "I must go up and evaluate him and take care of him." A patient appeared one day on the ward and told me "I was sorted out at Basingstoke," meaning "I was evaluated at Basingstoke and then transferred here with a diagnosis." The operating theater nurse would inquire when we were going to operate on a patient, and the senior registrar would respond, "Don't worry. We'll get it sorted." Lincoln would often walk into the operating theater and the senior registrar or I would stop and respond to a question. He would say, "Don't worry. Carry on.

Carry on." An expression I heard in the World War II movies, "Carry on" is still used occasionally, but perhaps only by those of Lincoln's generation.

The various professions and occupations had interesting descriptions. A "builder" is a construction worker. A "fitter" is a sort of plumber, and a "sewer" is one who sews. Of course a "sister" is a nurse, and a "porter" is an orderly. A maid in the UK is called "a woman who does for me" or "a daily" or "a cleaner"—never a housekeeper. A "Bobby" is a London policeman. A clerk is pronounced "clark" ("That Egyptian patient is a clark in Cairo."). A "publican" is one who owns a pub, and a "pensioner" is a retiree.

Certain expressions were rarely used in the States, such as "forename and surname," meaning first name and last name; "tick," meaning checkmark (e.g., "tick them off on the page"); "Hoovering," meaning vacuuming; "nackered," meaning tired (someone told me it meant specifically sexual exhaustion); "to sack," meaning to fire; "standing down," meaning resigning; "smart," meaning stylish; "queue," meaning line ("Your friend is waiting in the queue over there."); "ballux" and "pillux," the meanings of which I still don't know; "dodgy," meaning of questionable veracity; "rubbish," meaning trash (used as a noun or verb); "trousers and tunics" for pants and shirts; "braces" for suspenders (an Englishman does not wear suspenders!); "bespoke," meaning handmade; and "jumper," meaning sweater.

The British say "coach," meaning bus; "holiday" instead of vacation; "lift," meaning elevator; "elevator" instead of escalator; "diary," meaning schedule ("Before saying yes, let me check my diary."); "woolly," meaning unclear; "wally," meaning fool; and "randy," meaning a man interested in sex. "Bang on" and "crack on" seem to mean the same thing; I'm not sure what "crack off" meant. "Football" meant soccer; "flat" meant apartment; and "lorry" meant truck. A "bottom drawer" was the same thing as a hope chest for a young woman preparing for marriage. A "push bike" was a bicycle. "To knick" meant to steal.

Listening to Tony Desouza dictate a letter or operative report was interesting. "Naught" meant zero, "zed" was the letter z (Paul Peters gave me a popular map book of London called *A to Zed*), a "full stop" was a period, a "stroke" was a slash, and "inverted commas" were quotation marks. Desouza had the habit of saying "isn't it?" at the end of declarative sentences, and a favorite expression of his, as I mentioned before, was "bloody hell."

There were all sorts of names for the male human being, including chap, mate, bloke, and punter. "Cheers" was used interchangeably with "thanks," such that if you open the door for a man at a pub, he might say to you, "Cheers, mate." Only twice did I hear the expression "Cheerio," which is one of the relics from earlier generations, depicted in Hollywood movies of the English. The expression "ta," used for thanks, was said regularly by Paul Peters in the operating theater. A "fortnight" was used regularly to mean two weeks, and "stone" was used regularly to describe someone's weight. A stone is equal to 14 pounds, so one might say, "I weigh 12 stone." Lincoln sometimes used "score" for 20, as in, "This man does not need an operation. He has lived the Biblical three score and ten." An Englishman wouldn't say "I shall see you in two years." He would say "I will see you in two years' *time*."

The word "brilliant" had a wide context: "The weather was brilliant" or "You look brilliant." The nurse might say "The patient is doing well," and the senior registrar would respond, "Brilliant." The English also liked the expression "fair enough" owing, I'm sure, to their high regard for justice.

I had minor difficulty with the description of time early in the year. Someone would say "Be at the pub at half seven," and I did not know whether that meant 30 minutes before seven or 30 minutes after seven. It meant 7:30, and I was told that it is short for "half past seven." The British also read numbers differently. The telephone number "499–3662" would be read as "4 double 9, 3 double 6, 2." Unfamiliar with this technique of reading numbers, I occasionally had to ask my British friend to repeat a numerical sequence.

The language presented difficulties that were not insurmountable. But during my first week in London, if an Englishman had said to me—"Come by coach to my flat at half five. Take the lift to the fourth floor. The lady who does for me will let you in. I will set out the crockery and cutlery for you, together with a starter and a shepherd's pie. You will find a bespoke jumper in the closet if it is cold. Don't knick it. The fitter is coming in a fortnight, together with the mender. I wrote their surnames in my diary on the table. The fitter is a bit dodgy, and the mender is a wally. Feel free to sack him if he cannot sort out the problem. He weighs 19 stone, though, so you may need to call a bobby. Why don't you liaise with the other blokes in the building and go clubbing? Remember, no drink driving. Or you could pitch up and do some Hoovering in the flat. If the electricity goes out, you will find a torch in the closet next to my push bike. Don't worry—in one year's time, I shall return and we'll organize a meal together."—I would have thought we spoke different languages.

Certain words were also pronounced differently, such as "affluent," with the accent on the first syllable; "leisure," with a soft e; "vivacious," with a soft i; "good" as if it were spelled goot; "garage," with the accent on the first syllable; "recourse," with the accent on the second syllable. One English nurse seemed to enjoy correcting my colonial tongue. "Schedule" was pronounced "shejule." Various medical words were also pronounced in ways unusual to me: the beta in beta blockers had a long e, as did the e in trachea, with the second syllable accented. Carina did not have a long i.

Many subtleties of the language would take longer than one year to discern. Lincoln spoke the English language slightly differently, for example, than the registrars in surgery. He used expressions like "I would have thought that . . ." and "'Tis a pity," and "as you say," and "fortnight," and "stone" for weight. He never said "dodgy" or "mate" or "isnít it?" or "ta," expressions that are used often by the younger generation.

Lincoln admired what he called "BBC English"—the highbrow language of the newscasters of the British Broadcasting Company. They were chosen carefully, a highly educated people, Lincoln said. Regional accents of any kind were avoided. The broadcasters spoke the very best English. "Now the broadcasters of the BBC are chosen," he said, "specifically to exhibit a regional accent, in some misguided effort to get close to the people." Lincoln lamented this decline in standards.

During the year, high school students occasionally spent the day with us in the operating theater, as part of an educational program. A beautiful young woman from one of the prestigious London schools appeared one day above the ether screen. She asked very intelligent questions with an odd accent. It was as if there was no accent. Her vocabulary was rarified. I asked Lincoln with what accent she spoke, and he said, without hesitation, "Upper Class, BBC."

Michael Rigby, a pediatric cardiologist, told me once that the hiring of Professor Anderson at the Brompton in 1974 was controversial because he did not have the correct BBC accent or lack of accent. Rigby said that in those days, "everyone expected you to speak with BBC English." Several times during the year, Rigby expressed to me admiration for Lincoln as a surgeon, and Lincoln occasionally advised me to ask Rigby about various cultural questions, if he could not answer them himself.

Chapter 17

Harley Street and the Wellington

Lincoln carried on a private practice in addition to his National Health Service (NHS) responsibilities. Usually two days a week he went to either the Harley Street Clinic or the Wellington Hospital in London to operate on private patients. The Wellington Hospital was near the St. John's Wood tube station. Lincoln usually operated there on Monday mornings and Friday afternoons. The theater environment was quiet and efficient, and the operations usually went quickly.

I either first- or second-assisted Lincoln in these operations and enjoyed the experience. He had two regular assistants, Richard Angwin and Sayet Kosker, one of whom was usually present as well. Both men trained in cardiothoracic surgery in the UK but did not pursue career opportunities in the NHS. A friendly Englishman, Angwin rarely appeared in the second half of the year, because he was injured in a motorcycle accident. Originally from Turkey, Kosker usually opened the chest and took down the mammary artery, while I harvested the greater saphenous vein from the leg. After the case, I often rode back to Chelsea with Kosker in his BMW. He had a highly intelligent daughter who attended St. Paul's School, the most prestigious girls' school in London.

Lincoln remarked early in the year that if he needed a redo cardiac operation, he would want Kosker to open the chest. Reopening a chest was a challenging surgical task, and Lincoln believed it could not be taught. "I would let my Turkish assistant do a redo sternotomy on me," he said, "but I would not let it be done at the Brompton. Sir Magdi may have a Fellow from God-knows-where reopen a chest at the Brompton while he is still at Harefield. . . . I think the ability to reopen the sternum is a gift—either you have it or you don't."

On one occasion in the locker room at the Wellington, I ran into Alan Wood, a cardiothoracic surgeon from the London Chest Hospital. He regularly operated on private patients at the Wellington, assisted by the distinguished retired surgeon Matthew Paneth, who was a cardiothoracic surgeon at the Brompton Hospital for many years. Paneth would assist Wood by harvesting the greater saphenous vein during coronary bypass operations. I first met Wood on the airplane going to Dublin for the meeting of The Society of Cardiothoracic Surgeons of Great Britain and Ireland. We sat beside one another, and he was extremely talkative. A very busy cardiac surgeon, he operated twice a week at the London Chest Hospital in East London, and other days at various private hospitals. He had trained under Lincoln briefly and had had a difficult time.

Wood related the story of how he was obtaining written permission for an operation Lincoln planned on a child the next day. As the trainee, Wood was doing the paper work. He said that he was drawing a picture of the proposed operation for the parents of the child when Lincoln appeared at the door. Lincoln inquired what he was doing, then told Wood that his detailed explanation was inappropriate, that it would make matters worse. Wood, as he told it, replied that he refused to obtain written consent from the parents without explaining the operation in that way. Lincoln fired him immediately.

Wood introduced me to Paneth one evening, and we conversed briefly. That particular evening, Paneth had lost the key to his locker and was wandering around the Wellington operating theaters searching for it. Lincoln had spoken of him many times and was fond of telling one particular story. Apparently on social occasions, Paneth would often ask a woman, upon meeting her, "Has your husband left you yet?" (something like F. Scott Fitzgerald, who would typically ask a man to whom he was introduced, "Do you enjoy sleeping with your wife?"). On one occasion, that had indeed happened, and the woman broke down in tears.

When told that I worked for Lincoln, Paneth commented, "He is very good in congenital heart surgery." It was my intention to interview Paneth individually to learn more about the Brompton during the span of his long career there, but I never did. Upon leaving the Wellington, Paneth asked me whether I had heard of "Paneth cells." I said that I had indeed heard of them, but I did not remember where in the body they were! His ancestor, Josef Paneth, an Austrian physician (1857–1890), had first described these "Paneth cells" in the gastrointestinal tract.

Lincoln frequently spoke of Paneth, whose career as a consultant at the RBH overlapped Lincoln's. Paneth was extremely devoted to cardiothoracic surgery, according to Lincoln. "If he was not at the Brompton, he was out of England." He had two daughters to whom he was devoted and was currently involved with his grandchildren.

Lincoln commented that Paneth told him that "after a cardiac surgeon has done his first 500 heart operations, he may stop worrying about referrals. The pump has been primed." When I was in the library of the RBH studying for the oral part of my thoracic surgery boards, I came across a book on operative techniques in thoracic surgery, co-authored by Matthew Paneth and Peter Goldstraw. The book was simple and the illustrations clear. I found it helpful, though it was published some time ago.

On the Friday of my first week in London in August, I went to the Wellington. It was, as I remember, the only time during the entire year that Lincoln drove me to one of the private hospitals. Before leaving, he asked me to wear a coat and tie, not my white hospital coat. As we walked out of his office, he handed me his briefcase, which I carried to his car. As I was walking with him carrying his briefcase, I thought to myself, "This will be an interesting year."

That afternoon, Lincoln started a coronary bypass at about 3 p.m. and then moved to a second room, where he performed an aortic valve replacement, concluding both operations by 7 p.m. When he suspended the aortic wall with two pledgeted Prolene sutures to expose the valve, he commented, "Charles, this is the only important thing that I have to teach you about this operation. I have not changed my technique in 20 years." That technique of suspending the aortic walls with a pledgeted Prolene suture tacked to the chest wall proved to be a very useful method of exposing the aortic valve. Lincoln used a two-layer suture technique when closing the aortotomy. One of his frequent comments was, "I want these words tatooed on my chest: close the aortotomy in two layers."

On one Thursday morning in the fall, Lincoln phoned me from the Wellington Hospital and told me to report immediately to the intensive care unit. An adolescent girl, on whom he had performed a total cavopulmonary connection (TCPC) was deteriorating. I placed a chest tube in the patient, and Michael Scallan, the anesthetist, inserted some monitoring lines. I was then instructed to stay at the Wellington all day to look after her. Lincoln telephoned during the day to inquire with his usual brevity, about her condition. Fortunately, she improved, and I went home at 6 p.m. Congenital heart operations were rarely performed at the Wellington, which did not have the in-hospital expertise available at the RBH.

Lincoln often performed private congenital heart cases at the Harley Street Clinic, however. I enjoyed going to the Harley Street Clinic more than to the Wellington. It was a rather small hospital on Harley Street and, from the outside, did not appear to be a hospital. The reception area was like a living room in one's home, and the four operating theaters were downstairs. Marc de Leval, a pediatric cardiac surgeon from The Hospital for Sick Children on Great Ormond Street, regularly operated there.

Harley Street was notable for its "medical embassies." Most of the Arab countries, for example, had an office where private citizens of that country made arrangements for their medical care in London. Many of Lincoln's private patients were foreigners. Lincoln once said that "you can look around 360 degrees for one mile and the land is owned by one person." No doubt the rental fee for office space on Harley Street was high.

Both of the private hospitals—The Wellington and Harley Street—provided trays of sandwiches and fruit and cookies in the theater lounge areas. This was always a treat. The scrub suits at the Harley Street Clinic were "Carolina blue" in color, and I particularly liked them. Occasionally on a Saturday there, I would help Lincoln do coronary bypass operations. We usually enjoyed the peace and quiet of a Saturday morning in the private hospital more than the hustle and bustle of a weekday at the RBH.

Though Lincoln operated at three different hospitals, a conflict rarely arose, as far as I could tell. One morning when we were operating at the RBH, however, he received a call in the operating theater that his patient at the Harley Street Clinic was bleeding. Lincoln had performed a repair of coarctation of the aorta in an adult the day before, and bleeding through the chest drains mysteriously started that morning. Lincoln was beside himself with anxiety. He declared that he routinely called the private hospitals where he had patients to be sure they were okay in the morning, before starting an operation at the RBH. On this particular morning, however, he had not called Harley Street. By a stroke of luck, Lincoln's Turkish assistant, Kosker, was already headed to the Clinic, and he immediately reoperated on the patient, who recovered well.

Lincoln once remarked that Donald Ross was the first surgeon in London to carry on a private practice in cardiac surgery outside an NHS hospital. At the time, it was considered impossible to perform high technology medicine or surgery in a private hospital. Ross would operate on Saturdays at the Harley Street Clinic and elsewhere, and Lincoln often helped him in these operations. Ross designed several instruments, one of which was a metal atrial basket that one connected to the end of the venous tubing for cardiopulmonary bypass. The basket was inserted into the right atrium just as one would insert a plastic cannula for drainage. I expressed an interest in this basket, because I had never seen one before. While we were at the Wellington Hospital, Lincoln instructed a nurse to "find out how much the Ross basket costs, for Mr. Roberts." Although it seemed to drain the atrium extremely well, the basket was a bit cumbersome for me to insert because it was larger than the narrow cannulas I had placed at UNC.

Though Lincoln embraced certain techniques of Ross, he did not perform the "Ross Operation," replacement of the aortic valve with a pulmonary autograft. I think Lincoln viewed it as mutilating to the heart. The pulmonary valve had to be replaced, of course, with a cryopreserved homograft, which often calcified over the years.

The peak consultant salary during my year in London was about £65,000 per year. In addition to that, a consultant might have earned a "merit award," which provided an additional £21,770 for a B merit, £38,100 for an A merit, or £51,710 for an A+ merit award. Lincoln once remarked that he made £90,000 a year, including an A merit, but I may have misheard him. He made the remark that though he operated upon a high number of NHS patients, "I wouldn't do it if I did not have my private practice."

My salary of £500 per month (after taxes were removed from a £770 gross salary) was paid to me from his own pocket—what he called "soft money." He also paid his secretary in part from his own income. Lincoln charged about £80 per visit to his private consulting rooms. When he admitted a private patient for a coronary bypass operation at the RBH, a deposit of £15,000 was usually requested to cover the expense of the operation and hospital stay.

As I mentioned earlier, Lincoln had become a consultant at age 39, so he had been in practice nearly 23 years when I arrived in London. I suspect his personal expenses were not excessive, and he was frugal. He rarely ate out in restaurants because he considered them "too expensive." He always asked for tap water in restaurants because he thought the sparkling and still water that was sold was "a racket."

Lincoln had developed a certain resentment toward some surgeons at the RBH who carried on a large private practice at the RBH, to the apparent detriment of their NHS practice. During the year, there was a program at the RBH called the "Saturday Initiative," which was a weekly effort on Saturday to operate on patients on the NHS waiting list, to shorten that list. In Lincoln's view, the Saturday Initiative, which was promoted by the then Conservative Government, was a political ploy. He considered it hypocritical and refused to participate. The NHS patients should be operated on *during the week,* he believed, and private patients should be operated upon on Saturday or at other hospitals. It did not make sense to him to operate on private patients on a Tuesday or Thursday at the RBH, instead of NHS patients. The Saturday Initiative, of course, meant extra money to pay for the nurses and surgeons and assistants and anesthetists to work. Several times during the year, I helped surgeons in this program and was paid about £100 per case as an assistant. It was an opportunity to work with other consultants and earn money.

Lincoln was opposed to allocating the limited resources of the NHS toward the repair of certain congenital heart defects in certain children, rather than to a 60-year-old with angina pectoris, for example, who needed a coronary bypass. The older person "deserved it," in his view. Lincoln had little enthusiasm for repairing atrioventricular septal defects in children with Down's syndrome. My father had also at one time expressed the view that these children should not be operated on, whereas I think the majority of physicians and surgeons do so.

Lincoln had a somewhat humorous attitude about money. He once remarked in frustration, on a night when he was required to operate on an NHS patient, "There are only two reasons to operate after 6 p.m.: if you're getting paid and need the money or you're having a row with your wife, and neither applies in this case." One of the anesthetic registrars, Sanjay Guatama, had been a surgical house officer several years before on Lincoln's team. Lincoln paged him to his office one afternoon and told him to come in and sit down. After a long silence, Lincoln looked at him and said, "I am very . . . very . . . rich." After another long silence, he said, "Thank you," and Sanjay left the office. As I have remarked before, Lincoln was an expressive human being, and this anecdote does not surprise me.

Lincoln even liked to suggest that he was more wealthy than perhaps he was. At the end of an operation, he would tell a nurse, "Tell my secretary I shall be ready to depart in my Gulfstream [airplane] at eight." According to legend, while at the operating table at the end of a long day, Lincoln turned to the nurse and said, "Call my butler. Tell him to chill the champagne, warm the bath, and bring me a virgin." Lincoln would occasionally remark to me, "Charles when you become rich and own a Carribean island, you will invite me, I hope. Send your private airplane to pick me up."

Chapter 18

Moraes and Chauvoud

Several visiting surgeons and physicians appeared at Lincoln's door over the year. A cardiologist from India stayed at his home for a time in the spring, as did a surgeon from Brazil, Professor Carlos R. Moraes. In June, Lincoln invited Professor Sylvain Chauvoud from Paris to perform two operations at the RBH. During the visits of Moraes and Chauvoud, I was invited by Lincoln to join them at dinners he hosted in honor of each of them, which provided an opportunity to get to know them as well as Lincoln in a social setting.

After visiting Lincoln in London, Moraes went on to the March meeting of the Society of Cardiothoracic Surgeons of Great Britain and Ireland in Dublin, where I conversed with him at more length. Graduating in medicine in 1964, Moraes spent two more years in Recife, and then two years in Sao Paulo under Zerbini, the pioneer Brazilian cardiac surgeon, whose first assistant at the time was Jatene. Moraes then went to Europe for a year in 1969, staying primarily in London. Lincoln had just returned to the National Heart Hospital after his year in Boston, and the two surgeons became friends while working as senior registrars for Donald Ross, more than 20 years ago.

It was a time when Marion Ionescu was promoting the use of heart valve replacements with valves constructed from fascia lata taken from the patient's leg. Lincoln recalled what a horrible experience the two trainees had participating in that operation, which was later universally abandoned. The thigh from which the facia lata was harvested often developed a seroma, or fluid collection, which had to be drained. Lincoln recalled fashioning the new valve with the facia lata tissue on the back table, how the operation took all day. He remarked, "You would not buy a used car from Ionescu . . . . I mean, from an Anglo-Saxon point of view, your middle class Englishwoman would be told by her husband not to deal with him." According to Lincoln, "There was almost a mutiny among the registrars because results were so bad." Ross, the premier heart surgeon in the UK at the time, persisted in this effort, however, to the amazement of Lincoln. Ionescu's operation was supported by other established cardiac surgeons in the UK at the time.

Lincoln's relationship with Ross, according to Moraes, was sometimes strained, probably because Lincoln so disapproved of the facia lata heart valve that Ross was implanting. Moraes believed that Ross was not a strong supporter of Lincoln in his application to be a consultant at the Brompton. It was Shinebourne, the pediatric cardiologist, who desired Lincoln to be appointed. Moraes said that Waterston at The Hospital for Sick Children on Great Ormond Street was an important mentor for Lincoln.

After Lincoln came back from his two-week holiday in autumn in Recife, he remarked several times how "dry" the operative field was when Moraes operated. Lincoln said that the mediastinum looked "bloodless, almost cadaveric." Moraes said that he learned the importance of hemostasis from his mentor Zerbini, in Sao Paulo, who was meticulous, because blood products were not readily available then. Moraes said he took back no patients for postoperative bleeding in the last year.

The history of Recife influenced the course of North American history, in that Recife was invaded by the Dutch in the 17th century, and the Portugese drove them away. The fleeing Dutch then settled in what is now New York City (New Amsterdam) in 1624. It was not until 1664 that the British took over.

Moraes said he lived on a beautiful beach and arose daily at 5 a.m. After a one-hour walk along the ocean, he began work at the hospital at 7 a.m. He was in practice with his son, a former trainee of Lincoln and my immediate predecessor at the RBH. Moraes said that his son was a "different surgeon" after his year with Lincoln. Moraes wished to visit Chapel Hill on his next trip to the States, he said, and expressed an interest in further communication. He advised Lydia and me to consider Recife for our honeymoon. "Ask Lincoln about the beaches," he said.

I did a literature search on Moraes and found several interesting articles he wrote, particularly on the operative treatment of endomyocardial fibrosis, a disease seen more frequently in the tropics. Lincoln had an English patient with this disease, upon whom he was very reluctant to operate. The young man was severely disabled with breathlessness when Lincoln finally scheduled him for operation. Regrettably, the young man died of heart failure on the table. His was the only intraoperative death during the year.

Moraes spent the day at the RBH in March observing from above the ether screen in both theaters that Lincoln supervised. In one room, I assisted Lincoln in replacing a left-sided atrioventricular valve in a child who had recently undergone repair of an atrioventricular septal defect. Following that operation, I closed an atrial septal defect in a child using a pericardial patch. Lincoln appeared once above the ether screen. As he walked away toward the end of the operation, he said "5 out of 10." I was told that Lincoln was similarly graded by his mentors and followed their example of never giving a score above 5, which gave me some relief. I learned later that a former trainee of Lincoln now grades his registrars on the same scale: "Naught (zero) to 5 out of 10."

That evening, I attended a dinner in honor of Professor Moraes hosted by Lincoln and Karen Jurgens, with Elliot Shinebourne and his South American wife, Julene Carvalho, also a cardiologist. We met at 7:45 p.m. at Lincoln's home for champagne. I asked to see again the painting of his great-uncle who was killed in the Great War in 1918, and then we walked up to the informal sitting room, where Lincoln pulled a little book from the shelf. It was a small volume of letters and recollections of this young pilot, privately published by the young man's father. Lincoln had considered donating the book to the Imperial War Museum, but decided against it, as it would probably end up in a file cabinet.

We then took two taxis to the River Café on the Thames, where we had a delightful dinner. The restaurant was run by two women, one American and one English. One of the women was Ruthie Rogers, wife of the London-based contemporary architect William Rogers, whose offices were next door. We drank more champagne, then red and white wine, then dessert wines, and most of us enjoyed their effect. I sat between Lincoln and Shinebourne, and the conversation was delightful. I won't say that anyone became inebriated, but we came close.

Lincoln told the story of his last time in the restaurant with Karen. They had been seated at a table next to three "minders" (bodyguards), whose two charges enjoyed dinner at a table further away. Lincoln asked the waiter, "Why have you seated us beside the minders?" During our dinner, Shinebourne once turned toward Karen and asked, "Is it an English restaurant?" And Lincoln, mis-hearing, responded, "Yes, it is a Jewish restaurant," which broke us into laughter. I suggested to Lincoln that he come for two weeks to Charleston, and that I would arrange for him to stay at my mother's townhouse. He said, "I accept right now," adding that he desired to live in the States for a brief period again to experience the cultural differences.

Shinebourne had spent a year in San Francisco during his cardiology training. We talked at one point about the education of his son by his second wife. Lincoln was familiar with the school the child attended and with its headmaster. The headmaster apparently kept his office on the fifth floor of the building, and money did not necessarily ensure that one's child had a place at the school. The headmaster interviewed the parents before accepting the child and apparently noted their degree of breathlessness after climbing the five stories (there was no elevator). Shinebourne and his wife, both pediatric cardiologists, kept their child in this school from 8 a.m. until 5 p.m. most days of the week. On the exceptional days, the child was picked up by a caretaker. Lincoln seemed to admire the discipline of the school and said, "The future of England rests on this school," though not every student was stellar. Lincoln recalled one friend of his who received a postcard from his son, who was traveling with his class in Switzerland. The grammar and spelling were atrocious, and so the parents approached the headmaster, who responded, "Some children cannot be helped."

The visit by Professor Sylvain Chauvoud and his wife, Dominique, from Paris, was in July. Chauvoud worked with Alain Carpentier at The Hôpital Broussais. In contrast to the Brazilian Moraes, who is rather stout, the Frenchman Chauvoud was tall and slim. Lincoln paid his expenses to come to London and put up him and his wife at the Cranley Gardens Hotel in South Kensington. Chauvoud appeared the next morning with Lincoln in the catheterization laboratory to study the angiograms of the two patients with tricuspid atresia whom we had scheduled for operation. One patient was a little African child, and the other was a Greek woman in her twenties, a beautiful woman. Neither spoke English, neither had been operated on before, and both were blue because of their heart defects.

Lincoln had Marjan Jahangiri assist Chauvoud on the African child, and then I assisted him on the Greek woman. Chauvoud operated with great skill. He spoke fluent English, but, of course, he was not fluent with the English names of surgical instruments, though this did not hinder the progress of the operation in the least. The African child was out of the operating theater by noon, and the Greek woman was rolled in. When I opened the chest of this woman, I encountered torrential bleeding from collateral blood vessels throughout the sternal wall, such as I had never seen before. These mediastinal varicosities formed over the years because she was blue—her blood was not adequately oxygenated.

After I sawed through the sternum, the chest welled up with blood, and I thought for a moment that she would die, then and there, before Chauvoud even scrubbed in. While I was desperately stopping the bleeding, he casually glanced over the ether screen without saying a word. In a matter of minutes, I got the operative field dry, and the operation proceeded. Chauvoud once again operated with great skill, and both patients recovered well.

That evening, I attended the dinner in honor of Chauvoud at Lincoln's home on Pembroke Square, where we had the usual champagne and salmon appetizers. Chauvoud's wife Dominique was an ophthalmologist, tall and elegant in bearing. Her hair was black and drawn up behind her head. In contrast to most English women I met, she wore a fair amount of makeup. She rarely spoke, but when she did, her remarks were interesting.

Also present that evening was an English couple who were friends with Karen Jurgens. Lydia was in France, so I was the odd man out, so to speak. After champagne, we walked down the street to Stratford's, a French restaurant. Upon entering, Lincoln directed us where to sit. He positioned himself beside Dominique in one corner and me at the corner diagonally across the table beside Karen Jurgens. The conversation was lively, and I remarked to Lincoln the next week that each person was true to their country of origin. The English were English, the French were French, and the American was, I'm sure, American.

The Chauvouds recommended one or two hidden-away restaurants in Paris, and Lincoln kept saying, "Write it down, Charles." The subject of the American Revolution arose in conversation once, and the Englishman at the table remarked assuredly, "Of course the Americans learned from the French Revolution." Unable to restrain myself, I pointed out that the American Revolution occurred in 1776 and the French Revolution occurred 13 years later, in 1789, which brought laughter.

The Chauvouds admired Jefferson, which did not surprise me, as Jefferson was a Francophile to his dying day, July 4, 1826. He disliked England and would have the island sunk into the sea "were it not for its gardens." The Chauvouds had seen the recent movie, "Jefferson in Paris," starring Nick Nolte, which I had avoided. It involved Jefferson's relationship with his slave, Betty Hemings, which seemed to interest the Chauvouds. I walked back some ways toward the Cranley Gardens Hotel with the Chauvouds, then took a cab to my flat. I would see at a distance their tall, upright, slender forms walking briskly down the London sidewalk.

Lincoln made a point to write Chauvoud with a followup on the two patients that he operated upon. Whether Lincoln will ever do that specific operation on tricuspid atresia himself, I doubt. Inviting Chauvoud to the RBH at his own expense was an admirable gesture, particularly as Lincoln was essentially anti-French. "They have not gotten over the fact that the British and Americans saved them twice in two world wars," he said. The two patients were probably getting the best operation in the world, and the surgical trainees, Marjan and I, certainly benefited from Chauvoud's visit.

Lincoln interacted with French surgeons regularly at meetings in Europe and elsewhere. He remembered operating with Fontan years ago when the French surgeon came to the Brompton to help him perform a "Fontan procedure." I was assisting Lincoln at a coronary bypass when he said, "Fontan saw air, just like you, in the coronary arteries and declared 'It is air . . . it is air.'"

At a meeting at The Hospital for Sick Children on Great Ormond Street in the Fall, Lincoln introduced me and Paul Peters to LeCompte, another distinguished French surgeon. "There he is," Lincoln said, standing next to LeCompte, "the most innovative surgeon in Europe. All the secretaries know how to spell his name."

Chapter 19

Prague, Dublin, Hamburg

Apart from three visits back to the States during the year, I made three major trips abroad in Europe—Prague in October, and Dublin and Hamburg in March. As I mentioned before, I rarely left Chelsea to see England, the real England, let alone Europe. But these three trips were a taste of Europe, which I found much different than London.

The first trip abroad was to Prague, where the 1996 meeting of the European Society of Cardio-Thoracic Surgery was being held. On Saturday, October 5, Lydia and I flew from Heathrow to the Prague airport. We somehow managed to board the correct bus, which took us to the subway, which took us to the Don Giovanni Hotel, on the east side of town. A large heart sculpted in iron decorated the lobby. Our room had all modern conveniences. There was some confusion in my mind about what constituted a double room versus a single. In my experience in the States, all rooms had a bed large enough to accommodate two people, and the price was the same whether one or two people took the room. In Europe, the price of the room is higher if two people occupy it, i.e., a single room means a twin bed for one person.

Metro line A took us to the center of Prague. It was similar to London with regard to the height of the buildings and the ease of walking around downtown, but London is black and white and red with green parks, while Prague had winding cobblestone streets with yellow, pale, or mustard-colored buildings. The dominant entertainment in Prague was music. On every street corner, people were handing out advertisements for concerts, whereas in London, theater dominated. The two people Prague was most proud of were Mozart and Kafka. On Saturday night in the center of Prague, a small crowd had gathered around a young man seated on a chair playing a cello. All was quiet except for his music. Cars were kept from the center of town by barriers.

The subway stations in Prague were stark and enormous. Entry was dictated by an honor system. One voluntarily paid upon entering the subway station. In contrast to the tube in London, there were almost no advertisements on the walls of the stations. The underground in London is visually stimulating; in fact, I kept a wonderful collection of poetry called *Poems from the Underground* at my bedside for a month in the fall. This was an anthology of 162 poems that appeared at one time or another on walls in the London underground. I discovered Auden's "Song" in that book.

In general, the people of Prague appeared melancholic, though I may have misperceived their expressions, which appeared different from Londoners. The weather was hazy and the air dusty most of the four days. Our personal interactions with the Czechs were neutral, neither positive nor negative, except with taxi drivers, who routinely tried to overcharge us. One night we sought a ride from Mustek, the center of town, to the Don Giovanni Hotel and were quoted 600, then 400, then 350 crowns by three consecutive drivers parked in a row. In London, one never worried about being overcharged.

Saturday night Lydia and I, in the company of Paul Peters and George Stavros, dined at Parnuss, an expensive restaurant along the river. I was working with Paul Peters at the time on Lincoln's team, and George Stavros was also a surgical trainee at the RBH. The food was sumptuous and the setting relaxing. It reminded me of the Moscow restaurant in "Dr. Zhivago." I ate rabbit as an appetizer and fallow deer as the main course. Lydia remarked on the many pictures of deer on the wall in the restaurant in plain view as we ate deer! Stavros was from Greece originally, and Peters was from Manchester. The conversation flowed and was generally pleasant. We drank champagne, then dinner wine, then dessert wines. On Sunday night, Lydia and I dined at Restaurant Mucha, near Mustek. We drank a bottle of Czech red wine and enjoyed goulash, potato pancakes, and cabbage.

I attended the European Society of Cardio-Thoracic Surgery on Monday, Tuesday, and Wednesday morning. Andrea D'Armini, my close friend from Pavia, Italy, gave a presentation on Monday morning. At an Italian pharmaceutical company exhibit, we were offered delicious cheese and wine, over which we rejuvenated our friendship. I also had the honor to meet his chief in Pavia, Mario Viganó, about whom Andrea had frequently spoken.

We enjoyed dinner Monday night in the company of Dr. Peter J. K.

Starek, one of the two professors in the Division of Cardiothoracic Surgery in Chapel Hill. He was a superb coronary and valve surgeon and a gentleman. I had spent innumerable hours with him in the operating room at UNC and regarded him not only as my surgical teacher, but as a friend. Born in Czechoslovakia and raised in Iran (where his father built bridges as an engineering consultant), Starek came to Prague as a sort of homecoming. He still had relatives in the vicinity of Prague. Starek had arranged for Lydia and me to join him on a riverboat cruise down the Charles River, hosted by Medtronic, the early pacemaker company that is now a large corporation. The boat departed from Karl Square and took us within view of the Prague Castle. At our table of four was an articulate Frenchman who worked for Medtronic. He seemed to me an example of the so-called "corporate citizen" of the world, more so than a "national citizen."

Walking through the center of Prague on the way home, Lydia and I stopped at a nightclub to dance. Many men, as well as women, danced by themselves, which struck me as odd. A large movie screen at one end of the club showed something like an episode of "Wild Kingdom" involving predators and prey.

Tuesday night at the Prague Castle, which sits on the crest of a hill overlooking the Charles River, was most memorable. After champagne, hors d'oeuvres, and classical music in a large reception room, we entered Spanish Hall, which was enormous—high ceilings, chandeliers, yellow and white walls, and innumerable waiters and waitresses dressed in black. At our table, we sat with Drs. Starek and D'Armini, as well as the internationally known French surgeon Francis Fontan, after whom the Fontan operation is named.

Fontan informed Lydia and me that he was the first president of this particular surgical society. The food was unremarkable, but my conversation with Fontan was notable. He asked me to guess what country in the world he admires most. He quickly discounted the USA as "too young," and then said Italy, the "source of civilization." Fontan conducted a private practice in Bordeaux and had a chateau vineyard. He asked me if I thought I could distinguish between red and white wine when blindfolded. "You can't," he said. Even he, owner of a vineyard, said he could not do it.

Fontan had the most admiration for Carpentier among living French surgeons, and he held Kirklin of Alabama in great esteem. He said Kirklin did not show him or allow him to review the chapter on "Tricuspid Atresia—Fontan Operation" from the Kirklin and Barratt-Boyes book. Fontan asked me if I had read the Preface in the Kirklin and Barratt-Boyes book, in which the authors acknowledged the assistance of Fontan on a different chapter, *not* the chapter on the "Fontan operation." Fontan advised me to "be a better cardiologist than your cardiologist" and to keep writing, "if only for your family." Toward the end of dinner, he took my menu spontaneously and wrote several kind words to me above his signature. When Lydia and I arose to go to the reception area to dance after dinner, the music suddenly stopped. Fontan, still seated, remarked, "You two don't need music to dance."

In March I took two trips alone, as Lydia had not yet moved to London—first to Dublin and then to Hamburg. Lincoln had suggested that Tony Desouza and I attend the Society of Cardiothoracic Surgeons of Great Britain and Ireland, which was holding its annual spring meeting in Dublin on March 19–21. We left on a Wednesday morning and stayed at the Shelbourne Hotel, located on St. Stephen's Green, only three blocks from the meeting, which was held at the Royal College of Surgeons of Ireland.

Named after the 18th century British prime minister, Lord Shelbourne, the hotel was built to cater to the needs of the Anglo-Irish landed aristrocracy, who did not wish to hold on to their Dublin townhouses the whole year round. Lord Shelbourne had negotiated the peace settlement with the American Colonies in 1782. The English writer Thackeray, who stayed at the Shelbourne, wrote about the setting of the ground-floor window looking out on the Green, "A person with an allegorical turn might examine the entire country though this window." It was no wonder that Lincoln recommended it. One evening I attended a reception in the Constitution Room on the first floor, which overlooks the Green. In that room the first constitution of the Irish Free State was written in 1922.

From a medical standpoint, there were two highlights. Donald Ross gave the Honored Guest Lecture on Thursday, entitled "Journey through Cardiothoracic Surgery—the Early Days." He was introduced by David Wheatley, a fellow South African heart surgeon living in the UK. I was intrigued by Ross's talk, the first slide of which was a photograph of Christian Barnard, the South African who performed the first human heart transplant in the world in 1964. Christian Barnard and Donald Ross were classmates at Capetown, and each had achieved international fame in cardiac surgery.

Upon leaving South Africa, Ross trained at Bristol under Belsey, the general thoracic surgeon, who then recommended him to Brock, the pioneer British heart surgeon in London. In 1952, Ross went to Guy's Hospital and remained in London thereafter. Most of Ross's talk concerned Brock, whose career goal, according to Ross, was the operative correction of tetralogy of Fallot. He thought Brock was of the "prima donna era" of surgeons, a "Sauerbruch type" (famous German thoracic surgeon) who couldn't work as a team player. "His whole upbringing was that he was the boss." Ross emphasized that cardiothoracic surgery involves a team approach to be successful. Brock was obsessed with temperature, according to Ross, and kept the operating theaters overheated. He established the first ITU (intensive treatment unit) in the UK, similar to the ICU in the States. Brock apparently became thyrotoxic, went into atrial fibrillation, and was treated by thyroidectomy. Ross viewed surgery as "an art, not a trade, not a business, a calling."

The second highlight of the meeting was the Tudor Edwards Lecture delivered Friday morning by Peter Goldstraw, the renowned thoracic surgeon at the RBH. His talk was called "Advances in the Intrathoracic Evaluation of Lung Cancer." Goldstraw commented on the achievements in the operative treatment of lung cancer made by Arthur Tudor Edwards at the old Brompton. Every day, Goldstraw remarked, he walked past the wall of photographs of the former notable surgeons and anesthetists at the Brompton, and he wished that the glory days of general thoracic surgery (not cardiac surgery!) would come back to the RBH. He seemed determined to put the RBH back on an international stage in thoracic surgery. Goldstraw emphasized the importance of proper intraoperative staging of lung cancer, insisting that "the truth is there at the time of thoracotomy." He believed in systematic nodal dissection at any operation for lung cancer, that this was a habit which must be adopted.

The annual Dinner of the Society of Cardiothoracic Surgeons of Great Britain and Ireland was held at the IMMA Royal Hospital, Kilmainham, Dublin, on Thursday night. The reception room was right out of medieval times with its stone floors and candles. We moved into a dining hall, and I sat at a table with Tony Desouza. Vincent Young and Desouza won awards for the best scores in the UK on their cardiothoracic board examinations. I sat next to a woman whose father had worked 30 years with the BBC. I told her that Lincoln had witnessed a decline in the quality of the spoken English at the BBC over the years. She confirmed it and said that her father groaned over it in retirement.

For several hours each day in Dublin, I relaxed in the Lord Mayor's Lounge of the Shelbourne Hotel, sipping tea, reading, and writing an occasional letter. Having purchased several books during the five-day trip, I was constantly torn between walking the Dublin streets and reading in Lord Mayor's Lounge. My natural inclination to read kept me in chair much of the time, with: *The Famine Ships: the Irish Exodus to American 1846–51,* by Edward Laxton; *The Irish Nuns at Ypres: An Episode of the War,* by D. M. See; *Cheerio, Titan: the Friendship between George Bernard Shaw and Eileen and Sean O'Casey,* by Eileen O'Casey; *A Packet for Ezra Pound,* by William Butler Yeats, which was a marvelous find in one of the many Dublin bookstores; and all the newspapers I could get my hands on.

Vincent Young, the Irish senior registrar at the RBH, had gone to medical school at Trinity University, and he took me and several others on a walk through the campus. In one of those amazing coincidences, we discovered that we had a mutual friend, Dr. Karl Byrne, who attended Trinity University for medical school and was currently a general surgeon on the faculty at the Medical University of South Carolina. Byrne joined the faculty there when I was chief resident in General Surgery. We operated together frequently and became friends. Young knew him from his Trinity days, which, according to Young, were notorious. Everyone remembered Karl Byrne!

I saw more children in Dublin in one day than I saw in London in a month. There were always children in the lobby, in the lounge, on the streets as I walked—all Irish, often roaming freely. I mentioned this to the English woman at the dinner, and she coolly responded, "They have no birth control." My only regret in Ireland is that I did not see the countryside. I brought back a beautiful wool sweater.

Later in March, I went to Hamburg for the weekend to see Germany again, 15 years after my first visit. The weather was wonderful, the air cool and crisp. I climbed the Tower of Michael, the hallmark of Hamburg, and looked down upon the busy docks. The harbor of Hamburg was enormous, and there were several large ocean-going vessels in dock being repaired. The interior of the "Michael," with its great organ and pulpit, was beautiful.

A good part of the day was spent at the Kunsthalle, which housed a large collection of paintings. The gallery had very tastefully arranged the old paintings in rooms where one could spend hours. Adjacent to the old gallery was a new building with four floors of modern art. I found not one object of art appealing in this entire building, but perhaps the sensibilities this art required were out of my range. In the middle of the floor in one room, there was a pile of sand. In another room, there was a video of a bald man with his head bobbing in and out of the screen, saying "Work." I would take one room of paintings by Edvard Monk in the Kunsthalle for the entire collection of art in the new gallery.

Determined to eat a hearty German breakfast, I had a delicious omelet in the Schwanenwik, Café im Literaturhaus, one morning. It was a large room with large windows and high ceilings and heavy wooden tables with white tablecloths. Immediately adjacent to the café was a literary bookstore, specializing in poetry.

In the Atlantic Hotel over glasses of white wine, I started a fascinating book called *Regeneration,* which won the Booker Prize in England in 1995. It concerned the relationship of Sigfried Sasoon, the World War I poet who became a conscientious objector, and his psychiatrist in the Scottish Infirmary where Sasoon was sent. An admirer of the World War generations, Lincoln had introduced me to writings of the World War I poets, and I had purchased a copy of *Memoirs of an Infantry Officer* at Harrington Brothers on King's Road. A first edition copy and a rather expensive purchase, the memoir was fascinating. In my education in the States, I had given little attention to World War I, and did not know, for example, that the British Empire lost over 900,000 soldiers in that war. The figure is staggering when one compares it to the 670,000 deaths in the American Civil War.

Remembrance Day was a major event in the year in London. November 11 was set aside yearly in the UK to remember those lost in the World Wars of this century. Specifically, however, the day marked the end of hostilities in 1918—"at the eleventh hour of the eleventh day of the eleventh month." Older citizens sold red poppies to mark the day, and people of all ages wore them.

On television that week, an English girl in her twenties, hosting a show similar to MTV in the States, was wearing a red poppy. Would a woman of her generation do such a thing in the States? I thought not. Americans are so oriented toward the youth and the future that an act of remembering our fallen countrymen in wars past would generate limited enthusiasm now. The older and younger generations in the UK seemed more at ease with one another than in the States. They drink beer comfortably in the same pub. Lincoln bought the doctors on his team poppies to wear on our white coats during the week.

Returning to London by British Airways on Sunday, I had the uneasy thought that the Germanic and English people will never achieve a European union. The language barrier alone was staggering, and the difference in temperament was obvious to this American. Lincoln and I had many discussions about the European Community, and he preferred to view himself as a citizen, not of Europe, but of the *world*. He once remarked that when he observed Germans, even today (this generation), he saw in them the capacity to carry out another Holocaust. In contrast, Lincoln could not understand how the Japanese could perform such atrocities in World War II. Lincoln admired the Orient, I think, more than the Occident.

Chapter 20

Other British Surgeons

Professor Sir Magdi Yacoub appeared at Jane Somerville's Thursday afternoon conference on my first day of work. Lincoln had no operations that day, so I went to her conference for the first and only time. Somerville called Yacoub "my Pharaoh friend" because of his Egyptian birth, and the surgical trainees called him "the Prof." Somerville remarked to me at that meeting that Lincoln told her that complicated operations for *adults* with congenital heart disease were for "young surgeons."

By volunteering to assist him on two coronary bypasses one Saturday morning, I met Professor Sir Magdi Yacoub, who typically operated two days a week at the RBH, Wednesday the entire day and Thursday in the afternoon. The other times he operated at Harefield and Old Court Hospitals. I found him to be quiet and polite and easy to work with in the operating theater. In contrast to Lincoln, Yacoub enjoyed classical music in theater. His stereo system had been placed on a trolley, which was rolled into his room on those days when he operated at the RBH. His primary surgical interest at the RBH appeared to be aortic valve replacement with either a homograft or a pulmonary autograft (the latter operation first described by Ross). He was conducting a large trial comparing the two substitute valves, the updated results of which Francis Ferdinand presented at the American Association for Thoracic Surgery meeting in Washington, D.C., in May 1997.

Yacoub's registrar the first six months was Kevin Lachapelle, a French Canadian, and the second six months, Francis Ferdinand. Several days after working with Yacoub, I received from him in the mail a book called *Conjectures and Refutations: The Growth of Scientific Knowledge,* by Carl R. Popper, author of numerous books on scientific philosophy. Yacoub told me that he learned about Popper when he read his obituary in *The Times*. Popper's philosophy of seeking "the truth" appealed to Yacoub, who spoke of him several times during the year. The best way to reach the truth, Popper believed, was to try to disprove hypotheses—prove that they were false, not that they were true—the principle of falsification, Popper called it.

In February, I had lunch with Yacoub in the cafeteria between cases. I asked him about the arterial switch operation he reported in 1976 and his knowledge at the time of Jatene's work in Brazil. Yacoub asserted that he had no knowledge in 1976 that Jatene had done the arterial switch three months earlier. They were working "completely independently." The subject of Osler somehow came up, and Yacoub inquired who wrote the definitive biography of Osler. I told him the author was Harvey Cushing, and Yacoub requested that I make a note of it for him, which I did on a random piece of paper. Indeed Yacoub had what Osler called "imperturbability," meaning "coolness and presence of mind under all circumstances, calmness amid storm, clearness of judgment in moments of grave peril, immobility, impassiveness."

While working with Yacoub and John Pepper over the year, Ferdinand often referred favorably to his firm as the "academic team," in contrast to Lincoln's firm, which was "nonacademic" because Lincoln had no appointment at Imperial College School of Medicine. He was a freestanding "Consultant in Cardiothoracic Surgery." Yacoub was the British Heart Foundation Professor of Surgery and the Head of Cardiothoracic Surgery at Imperial College School of Medicine. The academic and nonacademic teams differed in no obvious way. With rare exception, neither team taught medical students. Teaching of trainees by the consultant, academic or nonacademic, depended on the personality of the consultant, not his title. The house officers and registrars rotated freely under academic and nonacademic consultants during the course of their training.

In October, I attended a course at Harefield Hospital on the homograft in valve replacement, directed by Yacoub. I met two American cardiac surgeons at this conference, one of whom was Bill Cornell, who headed a private practice group in Phoenix, Arizona. I happened to sit next to him on the coach going back to Sloane Square. Cornell was actually looking for a new member to join his private group, which was the largest in Arizona, he said, but I was, at the time, hoping to return to UNC. I learned that he knew well not only Dr. Wilcox in North Carolina, but also my father and mother from their Hopkins days. Cornell had gone to college and medical school at the University of North Carolina, then trained in surgery under Blalock at Hopkins. He told me that he did a classic Blalock-Taussig shunt (subclavian artery to pulmonary artery end-to-side anastomosis) as one of his first operations as a chief resident at Hopkins. Blalock kept peering over his shoulder asking if everything was okay. Cornell kept assuring him that all was well until the very end, when he suddenly realized that he had inverted, rather than everted, the back row of interrupted sutures. He was petrified, but Blalock told him not to worry.

I also met Gary Lofland, a congenital heart surgeon from Richmond, Virginia, who had trained at Duke, then joined the faculty at Medical College of Virginia. After a period of discontent, he entered private practice in the same city of Richmond. He described a harrowing tale of litigation that followed his departure from Medical College of Virginia. Apparently, Andrew Wechsler, the chairman of surgery, sued him for entering private practice in "close proximity" to the Medical College, his former employer. Lofland got the backing of Columbia, the owners of his new hospital, and the case finally dissolved. I remembered him from ten years before at Duke when he was the "super chief," and I was a fourth-year medical student from Emory doing a one-month "externship" at Duke in David Sabiston's Department of Surgery. Now involved with the large hospital corporation, Columbia, Lofland remarked that he might leave Richmond if Columbia were to buy George Washington University Medical Center. This never came to pass, as Columbia was outbid by another hospital corporation.

The other conference organized by Yacoub that I attended during the year was the 28th annual meeting in May of "Cardiac Surgery," presented by the Imperial College School of Medicine at the National Heart and Lung Institute in collaboration with the RBH. It was a two-day event, which I attended sporadically as time permitted being away from clinical duties. The conference also had live televised operations from across the street at the RBH. The most distinguished guest invited by Yacoub was Alain Carpentier, the famed mitral valve surgeon from France.

This was a big event for Frances Ferdinand, the other American fellow, because he assisted Carpentier in a mitral valve repair one afternoon. I happened to be operating next door to them that day, so I did not view the live operation with the audience, but Ferdinand made a tape of it and made a point of showing it to anyone who would watch at his flat on Neville Street! Ferdinand was so excited, he arranged to spend some time with Carpentier in France in 1998.

Lincoln found Carpentier "ill-mannered." Carpentier spent a good deal of time later in the conference going over aspects of his operation, and Lincoln, who had also attended sporadically, got up and left, explaining that Carpentier loved too much the sound of his own voice. By

May, I had come to know Lincoln better, and when I saw him get up from his seat near the front, I knew right away the reason. "I think I am allergic to Carpentier," he said later.

Lincoln and I were discussing aortic surgery once, and Hans Borst, the German surgeon, was mentioned. Lincoln described him as "a self-promoter. He is the Yacoub of Germany." Another time, I was conversing with Lincoln in his office when he picked up a piece of paper and folded it into a tube, saying, "Yacoub would take this and say 'We'll use it for the esophagus . . .' and there would be no one in England saying he couldn't."

One of the interesting facets of Yacoub was that he had an enormous research operation, in addition to his clinical work. At Harefield Hospital and also at the RBH, many people worked under his direction. Most of the senior registrars I had contact with at the RBH had worked at one time or another on a research project with Yacoub. I asked him once how he maintained his energy—did he sleep? He said that he required very little sleep and that he was able to sleep at odd times, for example in his chauffeured car from RBH to Harefield. His driver was a sub-Saharan African, from Somali I think.

Yacoub's energy was spread so thinly in so many areas that sometimes the consequences were bad. Ferdinand presented an abstract of Yacoub's surgical results at the meeting of The Society of Thoracic Surgeons in Washington in May. Normally, one prepares the full manuscript well ahead of the meeting date, and it is previewed by a "discussant" at the meeting. Ferdinand went to Washington with an unfinished manuscript, which he and Yacoub completed in a hotel room the day before his presentation. It had to be typed by a local service in the city. The discussant for the paper the next day was apparently disturbed when he was handed the paper moments before Ferdinand rose to speak. Another abstract at that same meeting in Washington had to be revised because the clinical data was inaccurate. Yacoub relies heavily, I suspect, on his worker-bees, who may need closer supervision at times.

Periodically, Yacoub would appear in the newspaper with Lady Diana, who sometimes gave her attention to the RBH. Yacoub permitted her in the operating theater to view a cardiac operation, and this was caught on camera. As I remember, her mask was slightly low or the bouffant did not completely cover her hair, and so Yacoub was criticized for compromising the sterility of the operation for her sheer entertainment.

At one point I was on duty in the evening in the hospital when one of Yacoub's patients in the recovery room suddenly arrested. Ferdinand happened to be standing by and immediately opened the chest. I joined him and we started cardiopulmonary bypass because the heart beat would not return. Yacoub arrived and thought the left anterior descending coronary artery had dissected, causing acute myocardial ischemia (lack of blood flow to a part of the heart muscle). I took out a segment of vein from the leg, and he and Ferdinand performed a coronary bypass. In time, the heart function returned and cardiopulmonary bypass was discontinued. Bleeding was a major problem in that patient during and after closure of the chest. I remember standing there as about 500 ml of blood drained out of the patient's chest in one hour, and Yacoub posed the question to me, "How much bleeding in one hour is an indication to reoperate?" I said, "250 ml" or some number thereabout. Yacoub said, "100 ml," smiling. Of course, that rule did not apparently apply to this patient, who did not undergo reoperation for several hours!

Ferdinand always complained about bleeding after cardiac surgery at the RBH. He firmly believed that British patients bled more than American patients. But even the senior registrars at the RBH always complained that patients bled more at the RBH than at the London Chest Hospital, on the east side of London. Whatever the case, reoperating for bleeding brought great shame to the surgeon. I had to reoperate a couple of times, and Desouza and Ferdinand never let me forget it. Desouza teased Ferdinand mercilessly about his bleeding complications. Whenever we would get an announcement for a conference on hemostasis (stopping bleeding), Desouza would place the paper on Ferdinand's desk with a note, suggesting that he attend. Yacoub performed a great number of cardiac *reoperations,* and Ferdinand always insisted that bleeding was less if he opened the chest rather than Yacoub, who used scalpel and scissors more than electrocautery.

Yacoub was married to a German woman, and they had a son and daughter. He always wore a dark blue suit, a light blue shirt, and a blue tie, though one weekend day he appeared at the RBH in a sweat suit, changing into the scrub suit to operate.

Yacoub was sued once during the year by a family whose child had sustained brain injury during an operation. The family argued that they were not informed of the risk of brain injury when they gave consent to the heart transplant in their child. As I remember, Yacoub admitted in court that he did not inform the parents of the risk of brain injury because the risk was less than 1%—and he won the case.

The other surgeon in the "academic department" with an appointment at the Imperial College of London University was John Pepper. Lincoln told me that Pepper's father was a distinguished Rolls Royce engineer in the UK. Pepper was probably the busiest adult cardiac surgeon at the RBH. He routinely saw all his patients on early morning rounds, often before 7 a.m. He also regularly operated on Saturday morning. In the aortic valve replacement trial comparing the homograft and autograft, he was the other major participant with Yacoub. Ferdinand considered him most like an American academic surgeon of all the British surgeons we met. Most of the trainees believed that Pepper would follow Yacoub as the next "Professor." Pepper was interested in teaching, and ran the 8 a.m. Wednesday morning conference. He had a hearty laugh and was always congenial. In the States, he would be easily qualified to head a department of surgery or a division of cardiothoracic surgery. He called me into his office before I left London to discuss my training experience at the RBH, which I described in positive terms.

Lincoln went to South Africa with Karen Jurgens for two weeks in April. While he was away, I took the opportunity to watch de Leval at the Harley Street Clinic on Tuesday, April 8. He did three operations, and I assisted on two of them. Lincoln had kindly called de Leval to obtain permission for me to observe him operate. As I mentioned earlier, Lincoln admired de Leval greatly. He called de Leval "a thinker." The surgical modification of the Fontan operation devised by de Leval was embraced by Lincoln, who called this modified Fontan operation the "de Leval procedure."

When Lincoln wanted an opinion about a child with congenital heart disease, he called de Leval. Though Lincoln did not believe in exercise ("It's unnatural") or rising early, he commented occasionally on de Leval's regimen, which was swimming laps every morning before dawn. Lincoln told the story of de Leval getting his Porsche stolen from his driveway in the early morning hours. The neighbor of de Leval apparently heard the car being started and driven off, but fell back to sleep, thinking it was de Leval going swimming.

The first operation I observed was a resection of a subaortic obstruction in a boy who had had three previous cardiovascular operations. The second operation was a left atrioventricular valve repair about 10 days after an atrioventricular septal defect repair. The third operation was a repair of a partial anomalous pulmonary venous connection. de Leval was assisted by an Italian female surgeon, 34 years of age, who was spending six months with him at the Harley Street Clinic. He also had trainees who worked exclusively at The Hospital for Sick Children.

The techniques de Leval used were very similar to those of Lincoln. He was organized and prepared for all three operations. After each one, he sketched his findings on the drapes to show me and the Italian assistant what he had done. I walked with him around the Clinic's ICU, where he had eight pediatric patients, a very busy private practice.

On a Sunday in early April, Lydia and I went to Birmingham, England, where I observed two surgeons at the Birmingham Children's Hospital: Mr. William Brawn and Mr. Babulal Sethia. Having heard a great deal about Brawn and having heard him speak at the Liverpool meeting with Lincoln in August, I was anxious to observe him operating. Lydia and I were taken to Birmingham by Tony Desouza's sister and her fiancé, who were returning to their home in Birmingham by car on the same day that we intended to take a train. We stayed at the Travelodge near the center of town, which was clean and inexpensive. Lydia spent all three days touring Birmingham, while I went to observe operations.

On Monday, April 14, at the Birmingham Children's Hospital, I watched Brawn perform a redo coarctation repair through a median sternotomy. In the afternoon, I went with his perfusionist to the Priory Hospital in Birmingham to watch Brawn carry out closure of a ventricular septal defect and insertion of a conduit between the right ventricle and pulmonary artery.

That evening, Lydia and I ate the traditional Balti Indian cuisine. Birmingham was a more attractive city than I had expected. The center of town had a large performing arts center and a lovely canal area with stores and restaurants. A considerable amount of money had been invested in downtown.

On Tuesday, I went to the Queen Elizabeth Hospital to observe Brawn again, this time performing a day-long operation. The patient was a young adult with pulmonary atresia and a ventricular septal defect. I was impressed by Brawn's stamina and focus at the operating table. Like Lincoln, he did not appear to move particularly fast, but there were no wasted movements. The operating theater was quiet. It was obvious why his clinical results were so good. At the Birmingham Children's Hospital, he had a videocamera attached to his headlight, so that one could watch the operation on the television screen in the room. The hospital routinely scheduled one case daily and left the afternoon open for urgent or unexpected cases.

On Wednesday, April 16, I watched Sethia repair the tetralogy of Fallot in a child at the Birmingham Children's Hospital. In conversation with him after the operation, he told me that the day before he had performed a Ross procedure and a first-stage Norwood procedure while I was across town watching Brawn. He recorded notes in a personal computer immediately following each operation, and wrote an index card on each case. This sort of detailed record is rare and admirable.

Chapter 21

Spring Visitors

On April 16, the day Lydia and I returned from Birmingham to London, John Clayton Randolph arrived from Little Rock, Arkansas, for a five-day visit. Because Lincoln was still on vacation in South Africa, Randolph and I had an opportunity to rejuvenate our friendship, which had been epistolary for more than a decade.

Raised in Little Rock, Randolph entered Vanderbilt University, where I met him in our sophomore year. He was carrying William Buckley's *God and Man at Yale,* outside reading, along with his regular course work. He made straight A's at Vanderbilt before returning to Arkansas to be among his close friends. He graduated from law school at The University of Arkansas, where he was editor-in-chief of its quarterly Law Journal. He entered a prestigious law firm in Little Rock, and we continued our friendship by correspondence.

Randolph was erudite and gentlemanly in manner, but he did not suffer fools lightly, particularly uninformed liberals and Yankees. He devoured books, knew history and literature, traveled widely in the world, loved the South, and was a devout Episcopalian. As I had remembered him, Randolph was tall and slender and perfectly groomed. His personal items were packed neatly, and one had the sense that he was tremendously well organized. We gave him the living room and opened up the futon as a bed. For most of his five days, he traveled outside of London, but we spent a full day walking and conversing together.

Randolph and I toured the Carlyle House at 24 Shane Row, where Thomas Carlyle lived in the early 19th century with his wife Jane. Author of a history of the French Revolution and a biography of Frederick the Great, as well as many other works, Carlyle was known to me for his belief that "history is biography." Sir William Osler also frequently quoted the following lines of Carlyle and lived by them:

> Our main business is not to see
> What lies dimly at a distance
> But to do what lies already at hand.

The hostess at the home showed Randolph and me the visitors book, in which the signature of Thomas Hardy appeared shortly after 1900.

We also walked to the statue of Sir Thomas More, who was executed in 1535 by Henry VIII for his refusal to acknowledge the legality of Henry's divorce and remarriage. The statue of Sir Thomas More was close to the gardens of the More House, near the Old Church where he worshiped. Randolph and I also walked through the National Army Museum on Royal Hospital Road. After a couple of beers in the early evening at the Anglicy Arms Pub, we joined Lydia for dinner at an Argentine steak house in Chelsea.

Randolph was determined to see Edinburgh, but his first attempt failed. The Irish Republican Army (IRA) was making bomb threats, one of which halted his train in the middle of England. The train returned to London, but Randolph kept his ticket and tried again successfully two days later. Full of admiration for the Scots because "they carved out a glorious civilization in an extreme climate," Randolph visited a chapel at the Edinburgh Castle that had established a relationship with his current church in Arkansas. Also determined to set foot in France, he took a bus to Dover and a ferry across the Channel. After briefly setting foot on French soil, he promptly returned to England. Why he was determined to do this, I do not know. He had been in France before.

One night Lydia, Randolph, and I went to the Blenheim Pub around the corner from our flat. Our Arkansas visitor soon found himself in the middle of a discussion about John F. Kennedy with a middle-aged, working-class, Northern Irish Catholic woman. She spoke with great admiration for Kennedy, and Randolph spoke with nothing but disdain. They bought each other a beer, but it was quite obvious that Randolph's reasoning had no influence upon her romantic opinion of Kennedy.

During his brief visit to London, Clay read *Birdsong,* the novel by Sebastian Falk. A stirring story set in the time of World War I, it received much acclaim in Britain. I had read about half of it, and Lydia the entire book. Randolph typically read one book at a time through to the end. This contrasted with my own reading style, which was to alternate reading several books at one time. I usually finished most of them, but some I put down, never to pick up again.

Also during Lincoln's absence, Lydia and I were visited by Mark S. Bleiweis, the first-year cardiothoracic surgical resident at UNC. As I mentioned earlier, Wilcox had an arrangement with Anderson for the first-year cardiothoracic resident to spend two or three weeks in Anderson's laboratory in London in the spring. The two residents before Bleiweis had not especially enjoyed London, for various reasons, and so I feared Bleiweis would have a similar experience. It seemed to me, however, that he enjoyed immensely his two weeks abroad. His wife, Jennifer, joined him for part of the time, and Lydia and I met them at Leicester Square just after they had seen *Les Misérables*. They came out of the theater quite moved by the play. After walking around Leicester Square and Picadilly Circus briefly, we returned to Cafe Lazeez in South Kensington. There we drank wine and listened to jazz and enjoyed great conversation.

One evening Lydia and I invited Bleiweis for spaghetti and salad, one of the few times Lydia and I entertained at our flat, which was so small we could barely fit three at the table. Bleiweis is Jewish, and his father was a Holocaust survivor. During my year in London, information was surfacing that much of the Nazi loot, including Jewish wealth, had been sent to Switzerland during the war. At the end of the war, very little of it had been returned to the deserving Jewish descendants. A great legal case had begun in the States against Switzerland in an attempt to regain the Jewish property, and Bleiweis was interested in the controversy. During the year, a Swiss Holocaust Fund was started with $103 million, with more expected. The fund was set up under intense international pressure and was intended to aid victims of the Nazis and their families.

Bleiweis spent one or two days in the operating theaters, observing Lincoln and Shore. Though he was interested in the possibility of coming to the UK after completing his training at UNC, I did not particularly encourage it for practical reasons. Bleiweis had a wife and two children. London is expensive and much easier to manage when one is single.

One day Bleiweis and I visited the Royal College of Surgeons and the Hunterian Museum. I toured the Hunterian Museum about three or four times during the year, and showed Bleiweis the plaque honoring the Philadelphia surgeon, Philip Syng Physick, donated by George Sheldon, the chairman of surgery at UNC. I was intrigued by Hunter's collection of paintings of American Indians. He collected paintings of people of different races in an age, of course, when there were no photographs.

After the Royal College of Surgeons visit, Bleiweis and I went to The Hospital for Sick Children on Great Ormond Street to look around. de Leval had requested that I furnish him with a slide for an upcoming talk, so I used that occasion to bring the slide to him. The slide was of an illustration in the paper that Lincoln and I wrote. Regrettably, we did not see de Leval, but I gave the slide to his secretary, and then Bleiweis and I walked around the hospital, visiting the chapel inside the hospital, as Lincoln had suggested. It was stunning, and the resident chaplain kindly gave us a tour.

Bleiweis and I then went to the "Old Operating Theater and Herb Garret," located in the roof of the 18th century Church of St. Thomas near London Bridge. It dates from 1821 and was part of St. Thomas Hospital before it closed in 1862 and moved to Lambeth. The theater that we toured witnessed the advent of anesthesia in 1846 and was closed just three years before Lister began his experiments in antiseptic surgery. The motto that appears on the wall in the old operating theater is "Miseratione non Mercede," which means "from compassion, not for gain." Painted on another board on the wall were the theater regulations:

Regulations for this theatre
Apprentices and the Dressers of the
surgeon who operates are to stand
round
the Table. The Dressers of the other
surgeons are to occupy the three front
Rows. The Surgeons' Pupils are to take
their places in the Rows above.
Visitors are admitted by permission of
the Surgeon who operates.
George Chandler
Benjamin Travers
Joseph Henry Green
1821

Florence Nightingale founded her School of Nursing at the old St. Thomas Hospital in 1860 and advised on the hospital's subsequent move to Lambeth. It was thought that the original hospital was founded in the year 1106 and was renamed after London's favorite saint, Thomas Becket, in 1173. After the Great London Fire, it was rebuilt in 1215 to the east of Long Southwark, now Borough High Street, where the air was said to be sweeter. It remained on this site for 650 years.

Bleiweis and I walked down the street to see Guy's Hospital, which was built alongside St. Thomas's. In 1726, the first patients were admitted to Guy's Hospital, which was designed to admit the so-called "incurables" that St. Thomas's refused to accept. It soon developed into a general hospital. Sir Thomas Guy, a printer and publisher, is buried inside the hospital chapel, constructed in the central entrance.

In May, Lydia and I were visited by my father and older brother Clifford for five days. They flew in together from Atlanta, and I arranged for them to stay at the Cranley Gardens Hotel near the Pelham Hotel, where my father had previously stayed. On the night of their arrival, Lydia and I joined them at Hilliard's Restaurant on Old Brompton Road for an elegant dinner. Lydia then went to Scotland for three days with Leslie Jeng, and I joined my father and Clifford for much of their visit.

On their first full day in the UK, they went to Greenwich by boat. A book had recently appeared on the determination of longitude on the globe and its implications in sea navigation. My father bought a compass and seemed to ask everyone he met whether they knew how it worked, including three men at the Cranley Gardens bar, which sparked a lively conversation. On Saturday morning, I assisted Lincoln in repairing the tetralogy of Fallot in a child, while my father and Cliff toured London. They went to the Portrait Gallery and then saw a play called *The Fix,* which had to do with British politics.

On Saturday evening, my father hosted a dinner in honor of Lincoln. I invited Francis Ferdinand, Tony Desouza and his wife Sarah, and of course Lincoln and Karen Jurgens. Because Leslie and Lydia were in Scotland, males predominated; nevertheless, we enjoyed the evening. Lincoln invited us to his home for champagne and salmon before dinner. We then dined at the Bombay Brasserie on Gloucester Road, the Indian restaurant, where the food was quite good. I was pleased that my father had treated Lincoln to dinner, as Lincoln had so kindly invited me on several occasions. My father sat at one end of the table and Lincoln at the other. Desouza and I sat beside my father, and Clifford and Ferdinand sat beside Lincoln.

On Sunday, I assisted Lincoln on a very difficult case involving partial anomalous pulmonary venous return in a child. That afternoon, I joined Clifford and my father at the Apsley House, which was Wellington's home. Later that day, we went to the Museum of London, then had dinner in Chinatown at a restaurant called Fung Shing. On Monday, I went with them to the National Gallery, where Clifford noticed a wonderful painting of a physician at his desk with a book he had written on nutrition. He was apparently one of the first physicians to write a treatise on the subject, and so my father took down all the information.

One of my favorite paintings in the National Gallery was the portrait of Bannistre Tarleton by Sir Joshua Reynolds in the front hall. Tarleton commanded the British Legion in 1780 at the Battle of Cowpens in South Carolina, the worst British defeat between Saratoga and Yorktown. It was said that Tarleton lost the battle that lost the campaign that lost the war that lost the American Colonies. My other favorite painting at the National Gallery was "Young Man with a Skull," by Franz Hals. Holding a skull was in the Netherland tradition in portraiture, the skull being a "vanitas," a reminder of the vanity of life and the certainty of death.

On Monday evening, we dined at a French restaurant called La Brasserie on Fulham Road, where I had been with Carrita and my father during their earlier visit. My father and Clifford then went to see a play called *Buddy,* based on the life story of Buddy Holly.

Tuesday was a bank holiday, so I joined my father and brother in seeing the Bank of England museum, Dr. Johnson's home, and St. Paul's Cathedral. The museum at the Bank of England was fascinating. In 1694, the bank was founded during the reign of William and Mary (1688–1694). In 1946, it was nationalized, and in 1997, during my year in London, it was returned to the private sector. The year 1816 (one year after the Battle of Waterloo) was a major year in the history of the Bank of England because the gold standard was established. In the Gordon riots, which involved a conflict between Protestants and Catholics on June 6, 1780, the bank was attacked by a mob. Boswell wrote of this event in his life of Samuel Johnson.

On Tuesday night, Francis Ferdinand and John Pepper, the consultant academic surgeon, had arranged a dinner for my father at Dan's Restaurant, across the street from the RBH. The senior registrars in surgery were invited, as well as the consultants. Lincoln attended, and so did Derek Gibson, the cardiologist. There was a brief question/answer period, during which Francis Ferdinand directed several questions about medical editing to my father, who was the editor of *The American Journal of Cardiology.*

The evening went rather well, and my father had planned to speak at the Cardiac Surgical Conference on Wednesday morning. This had been arranged rather hastily, and my father never actually read the correspondence from Ferdinand until he finally returned to Dallas. The talk was to be at 8 a.m., and my father was to take a waiting taxi to Heathrow at 9:15 a.m, thinking that his flight departed at 11 a.m. When I arrived for dinner at Dan's on Tuesday night, my father said that his flight to Norway had been changed by his Norwegian hosts and that he would be leaving Heathrow earlier—so his talk on Wednesday morning had to be canceled. This was rather embarrassing to my father, who had missed only three speaking engagements in his 40-year career. On one occasion, he was snowed in at home in Maryland and could not get transportation to the airport. On another occasion, he was too ill to make the trip. And the third instance was this one at the RBH.

Chapter 22

Lincoln and Kirklin

Lincoln spoke of John Kirklin of Alabama with more frequency and higher esteem than any other surgeon in the world. During my first month in London, I recorded in my diary regularly that he mentioned Kirklin. He even imitated his speech occasionally; at any rate, I think it was Kirklin he was imitating when he said "ree . . warm" ever so softly at operation, so that only Victor, the perfusionist, whose ear was trained, knew that he was saying "rewarm" the patient. Lincoln also repeated a remark by Kirklin on operations in the elderly: "It is no different than operating on younger people, *if you can stop the bleeding*."

Lincoln and Kirklin appear to have interacted on two important occasions during Lincoln's career. The first was in 1982, when Kirklin visited Lincoln for a week at the old Brompton on Fulham Road. Kirklin came with the intention of observing an arterial switch operation for transposition of the great arteries, in which the pulmonary artery arises from the left ventricle, and the aorta arises from the right ventricle (Jatene in Brazil and Yacoub in the UK had performed the operation successfully only three months apart in 1976). For years Lincoln had performed a Mustard operation (atrial switch) for transposition, but eventually he embraced the new operation and was regularly performing it. Despite an irritating cough from an upper respiratory tract infection, Lincoln performed four operations that day, while Kirklin observed motionless above the ether screen.

In 1985, Lincoln was invited by Kirklin to Birmingham, Alabama, to speak on the arterial switch operation. Lincoln stayed at Kirklin's home during the visit and remembered certain details. Kirklin rose early and was in theater by 7 a.m. "Here was one of the world's greatest surgeons seated in a chair performing an arterial cutdown in the wrist *before* the operation." He watched Kirklin at the foot of the operating table align the patient properly before draping. Lincoln recalled amusingly that he was in a sterile gown observing the operation behind Kirklin when a nurse accused him of "breaking sterility"$—his gown had inadvertently touched a non-sterile pole. He was re-gowned, only to be accused by the same nurse of breaking sterility again in the same manner.

Lincoln was impressed by the number of beautiful women in a Birmingham restaurant, saying, "The Southern Belle as a social type exists. Al Pacifico made reservations for me at a restaurant in Birmingham. He couldn't attend, so I sat by myself and watched one beautiful woman after another enter. I was amazed. There is no greater truism than the existence of the Southern Belle." When we had a late start one morning at the RBH, Lincoln remarked that "Pacifico would have probably done four operations before breakfast."

Lincoln once wrote Kirklin to ask advice on "taking down" or ligating a Potts' shunt, a connection created surgically between the descending thoracic aorta and the left pulmonary artery. Kirklin responded that "it was relatively easy" and offered a brief description of the technique. Simultaneously, Lincoln had written Farouk Idriss in Chicago, who responded with a very detailed 12-step technique, which was successful, according to Lincoln, "only if each and every step was followed perfectly."

Lincoln involved me in one issue concerning Kirklin in the fall. When he received the program for the American Association for Thoracic Surgery meeting in April in Washington, D.C., Lincoln noticed that the lead abstract concerned complications after the arterial switch operation. The authors included William Williams from the University of Toronto and John Kirklin and Eugene Blackstone from the University of Alabama.

In the early 1990s, Lincoln and Williams had combined their results of the arterial switch operation in an effort to determine the incidence of right ventricular outflow tract obstruction after the operation, which appeared to be the most common postoperative problem. The incidence of that complication at Toronto and the RBH was similar. Lincoln and Williams combined their results, prepared a manuscript, and submitted it for publication in the *Journal of Thoracic and Cardiovascular Surgery,* which was then edited by Kirklin. The article was sent back to Williams for revision; and then, for some reason unclear to Lincoln, the revision process was halted. Williams appeared to have abandoned the project, and Lincoln did not aggressively seek an explanation.

Now, a few years later, Lincoln was reading an abstract by Williams to be presented at the American Association for Thoracic

Surgery, which must have included the same data from their earlier collaborative attempt. Lincoln seemed to feel misused by this sudden appearance of data similar to that which he had previously written up in manuscript form with Williams. He asked me into his office several times over a two-week period to discuss it. I was sort of "a sounding board." First Lincoln wrote Williams to express his surprise and to request a copy of the manuscript. In a reply to Lincoln, Williams offered no explanation as to why he had abandoned their earlier collaborative manuscript.

Lincoln also wrote to Kirklin to ask him whether he recalled the manuscript submitted by Williams and Lincoln to the *Journal of Thoracic and Cardiovascular Surgery* a few years before. Kirklin responded that all the manuscripts submitted and not published had been destroyed, but that he would furnish Lincoln with a copy of the new Williams manuscript when it was available. Both of the letters—from Williams and from Kirklin—were friendly, but neither was satisfying, in that Lincoln still never understood why his manuscript with Williams on precisely the same subject had been abandoned. Lincoln wrote many articles during his training and consultant years, but I am sure he had some regret that he did not pursue publication of this particular manuscript more aggressively at the time that it was abandoned.

Chapter 23

The Bristol Affair

My first exposure to the medicolegal situation in Bristol, England, was on Wednesday, March 19, when I read in the *Express* newspaper an article called "Heart Surgeon's Grim Toll of Tragedy," and the subheading was "Top Surgeon Quits after Baby Deaths." There was a picture of a surgeon named James Wisheart adjacent to the title. The first two paragraphs read, "Adults who had open heart operations by a top surgeon were four times more likely to die than with other specialists, it was revealed yesterday. James Wisheart's mortality figures were contained in a damning report into the 59-year-old surgeon." The fourth paragraph read, "The surgeon, who announced his retirement on Monday, stopped operating on children in 1995, when it emerged 9 of 13 babies he had performed open heart surgery on had died." I read this article on the way to Ireland and thought little of it until Lincoln called me into his office to discuss the subject later.

In 1995, the United Bristol Health Care NHS Trust authorities ordered a review of heart surgery at Bristol. The review of adult operations between January 1993 and November 1995 revealed a 12.2% mortality rate in coronary artery bypass grafting by Wisheart. A separate review was carried out of pediatric cardiac surgical cases, and it was this pediatric review for which Lincoln's opinion was sought.

A document called "Report in Respect of the General Medical Council/Bristol Pediatric Cardiac Surgical Case" was sent to Lincoln for an opinion by the lawyers of the two defendants, Wisheart and Janardan Dhasmana. The report was written by William J. Brawn, the prominent pediatric cardiac surgeon at Birmingham Children's Hospital, whom I had visited in April. Brawn, who had been a consultant for 17 years, the last nine of which had been spent at the Birmingham Children's Hospital, was asked to review the pediatric cardiac operative results at Bristol. In his conclusion, Brawn stated that "in the majority of aspects, the care for patients was good, in particular as regards the majority of the surgical program."

Brawn identified two operations, however, for which the results were suspect. The first was repair of atrioventricular septal defects performed by Wisheart, and the second was arterial switch operations performed by Dhasmana. The 36-page document, dated February 27, 1997, came down hard on these two surgeons. The attorneys for the two defendants sent the document to Lincoln, asking whether he would be willing to testify in defense of the two surgeons. For my education, I think, Lincoln asked me to review the document and express an opinion.

The document indicated that nine of 15 children operated upon by Wisheart for atrioventricular septal defect between 1990 and 1994 had died. After the twelfth operation on May 6, 1993, six children had died. The next three children died, as well. In the arterial switch operations by Dhasmana, 17 (45%) of 38 children died over a seven-year period, from 1988 to 1995. In particular, nine of 13 neonates died, and eight of 25 older babies died. Brawn's two concluding paragraphs were reasonable:

> I think there should be compulsory internal audit of surgical cases and catheter interventional procedures with reports being externally assessed. This should be a prerequisite for all centers carrying out congenital heart surgery in the country. There must also be a central coordinating body—perhaps the British Pediatric Cardiac Association or one of the Royal Colleges. This audit should be externally assessed and reviewed, with the results made freely available to all parties concerned, including parents, the General Medical Council, and other professional groups. It should be on an operator-named basis, rather than on an institutional basis.
>
> In addition, there should be nationally agreed guidelines as to acceptable mortality. I think morbidity is difficult to judge, but certainly 30-day mortality rates should be freely available to all professionals involved. This may identify procedures which are not being performed well in some less experienced units and lead to a greater acceptance that patients can be referred to centers where there is more expertise.

Lincoln and I discussed at some length his response to the attorneys. Michael Rigby, a pediatric cardiologist at the RBH, had also reviewed the Bristol cases and expressed the opinion that the pediatric cardiologists were also at fault for referring children too late for operation for repair of atrioventricular septal defect.

Ultimately, Lincoln declined to testify for the defense because he found the sheer mortality figures too high to support. He voluntarily offered his service, however, as a "sounding board" for the defense attorneys should questions arise during the case. He was initially hopeful, I think, that he might be able to come to the defense of both surgeons, and he appeared to struggle to formulate a defense for them.

I asked my father by telephone for his opinion in the matter, and he also thought it would be fruitless for Lincoln to embroil himself in this matter. My father had observed a most unfortunate medicolegal situation involving his friend Dean Mason, the editor of the *American Heart Journal,* in California. He considered Dean Mason to be perhaps the smartest man he had ever known, and this long term medicolegal issue that involved him at the University of California at San Diego depleted his energy.

Lincoln admired Brawn as a congenital heart surgeon. Brawn had come down to the RBH in the past and operated, and Lincoln had observed him. Brawn's operative results were excellent. It was the idealism of Brawn that concerned Lincoln. At one point while we were operating, out of the blue Lincoln said, "I wonder if he is religious." I said, "You mean Brawn?" He said, "Yes."

On another occasion, after the meeting in Liverpool when Lincoln and Brawn were present, Lincoln remarked, "Bill Brawn is in his own world." During the conference, a child with no intrapericardial pulmonary arteries was presented to the four distinguished pediatric cardiac surgeons present. Lincoln said that he would not attempt a total correction, but rather do a right modified Blalock-Taussig shunt. Brawn expressed the view openly in the conference that that was an unsatisfactory option for the child; instead, one should attempt a total correction of this malformation. It seemed to me a case of an older, experienced surgeon pitted against a younger, idealistic—though extremely talented—surgeon.

From time to time during my last six months, I asked Lincoln how the Bristol affair was going, but the hearing was delayed until the fall of 1997, so that when I left in July, it was still unresolved. Ultimately, the physician in charge of the United Bristol Healthcare Trust, Mr. John Roylance, was also targeted by the General Medical Council for not adequately addressing the high surgical mortality when it was initially brought to his attention.

Several articles in the June 6, 1998 issue of the *British Medical Journal* were devoted to the Bristol situation. Rudolph Klein of the University of Bath wrote:

> The case of the three doctors in Bristol represents a landmark in the history of the self regulation of the medical profession in the United Kingdom in terms of its length, its salience in the eyes of the public, and the issues it has raised. It has stretched over eight months and involved more than 60 days of hearings before the General Medical Council—probably the most extended and expensive case in the history of the GMC. It is the stuff of which headlines are made; it is highly charged emotionally since it concerns the deaths of children after heart operations. And it has provided a test case for the GMC's policy of seeking to ensure that all members of the profession accept their collective responsibility for maintaining standards and practising within the limits of their competence.

The ruling by the General Medical Council finally came in July 1998. The former chief executive Dr. John Roylance and the former surgeon Mr. James Wisheart were "struck off" the medical register, even though both had already retired. Mr. Janardan Dhasmana was allowed to stay on the medical register, but prohibited from performing pediatric cardiac surgery for at least three years. The Bristol affair was considered one of the biggest tests in the 140-year history of the General Medical Council, and its ruling prompted a flurry of editorials in lay and medical publications.

Chapter 24

Medicolegal Matters

During the year, Lincoln discussed several medicolegal cases that came across his desk. Apparently not one of these was directed at him, but he was asked to provide an expert opinion. Early after my arrival, he was reviewing a court case in which the plaintiff argued that because the surgeon did not evacuate air from the left atrial appendage at the end of the operation, the child suffered a stroke from an air embolus. For several weeks, he periodically brought up this case, saying, "I warn you. I always invaginate the left atrial appendage with my fifth left finger to expel air." It was typical of Lincoln to instruct his trainees. Teaching came naturally to him.

In the fall, shortly before his trip to Brazil, he was preparing a talk that he humorously called "The Truth." To be delivered to a Brazilian medical audience, it dealt with malpractice litigation. He admitted, however, that "my talk on the truth is probably inappropriate for a Brazilian audience, who have so little malpractice litigation."

Lincoln was particularly specific and clear, as I mentioned earlier, in delineating the risks of surgery to the parents of children, and would write these risks beside the name of the operation on the written consent form. He mentioned one occasion when he was co-defendant in a court case with Elliot Shinebourne, the pediatrician. I do not recall the specifics of the case, but while on the stand answering questions, the judge accused him of being "dismissive." While recollecting this episode in the operating theater, he asked the nurse Faye Too to retrieve the dictionary from his office to look up the meaning of "dismissive." (To be "dismissive" means to be without attention to or serious consideration for the matter at hand.) Lincoln was fascinated with words, and it was not uncommon for him to call for the dictionary during an operation.

Another phrase we heard one day prompted Lincoln to call for the dictionary: "Light-weights, lackeys, and lickspittle." A lackey is a camp follower, and a lickspittle, we learned, was "an abject parasite; a toady." This three-part phrase was used in London in days of old, but we liked the phrase "an abject parasite."

One unfortunate episode prompted Lincoln to call a meeting of the members of his team. A new pediatric intensive care unit specialist, Dr. Dan Penny, was hired as a consultant from Melbourne, Australia, where he had last trained. He had also trained for a time at the RBH with Andrew Redington, and so he was familiar with the institution. For some reason, Lincoln and Penny did not see eye to eye on certain patient care issues, and Lincoln expressed his views very strongly against the management dictated by Penny.

On two occasions, Lincoln openly criticized the management of the children by Penny, expressing his opinion forcefully in the presence of Penny's trainees. Parents of patients in the ICU apparently overheard the comments. On both occasions, Penny apparently expressed his objection to Lincoln immediately, asking him not to criticize his management publicly.

Present at neither episode, I cannot offer the details. I had met Penny shortly after his arrival and was on friendly terms with him, when he expressed his chagrin to me about the two episodes. The second episode concerned the fact that one of Lincoln's operations was canceled because of a shortage of nurses or beds in the ICU. A patient of Darryl Shore, in contrast, was kept on the operating theater list that day. Lincoln accused Penny of canceling his cases in favor of Shore's. By Penny's account, when he objected to that accusation, Karen Jurgens chimed in to support Lincoln's side, which particularly irritated Penny. He analyzed a number of recent cancellations and found that the frequency of cancellations was similar among Shore's and Lincoln's patients. This data was conveyed by Penny in a memorandum to Lincoln, in which he described the two episodes as "your recent outbursts."

Penny also registered a written complaint with Shore, who was the administrative clinical director of the pediatric unit at the RBH. Instead of dealing with the matter at his level, Shore escalated it to the hospital administrative level.

One morning, two administrators appeared in Lincoln's office to discuss the situation. In so many words, they said that if the problem could not be resolved, they would have to take it to a higher authority in government. Of course the destructive potential for Lincoln was high. He called us into the office and told us all the details of these events so that "we would squelch any rumors that might arise." I do not know whether Lincoln formally apologized to Penny or how the issue was finally resolved. Lincoln continued to go to the Pediatric ICU on a daily basis, but he did not speak to Penny if he could avoid it, remarking, "I have gotten along fine without him for 23 years, and I can continue to do so until I retire."

This series of events was an education to me, showing that a matter not concerning one's competency in medical care, but rather one's interpersonal relationships, can severely compromise one professionally. It reminded me of an episode that occurred early after my father started a job. He met with the chairman of medicine to discuss the possibility of assuming control of training in cardiology. The discussion became heated, and my father raised his voice. The consequences were disastrous, and my father has brought up the episode to me on several occasions as an example of what not to do.

Chapter 25

Home and Back

In June, I returned to the States for 10 days, my third and final visit from London. I flew into Chicago on June 5, checked in at the Omni Hotel, and on Saturday morning, took the oral portion (Part 2) of the American Board of Thoracic Surgery Examination. The test was not particularly difficult. I had four examiners during the 8 a.m. to 10 a.m. session, each examiner questioning me for 30 minutes in a separate hotel room. Each examiner presented two patient scenarios, about 15 minutes each. I was given a badge with a number to pin on my lapel. No names were exchanged in the interviews.

The first examiner was Floyd Loop, from the Cleveland Clinic, who presented a child with a ventricular septal defect and then a young adult who needed an aortic valve replacement. Repair of the ventricular septal defect I described easily. For the aortic valve replacement I described using a homograft, to avoid anticoagulation. Though I had never performed the operation, I had assisted Yacoub and also observed him several times doing the operation. In my view, it was the right procedure for the patient, and I had certainly memorized how to do it. Loop was courteous, and the interview went well. He asked me if I would take any special measures because the aortic valve replacement was a *reoperation.* "I would give aprotinin," I said, and that sparked his interest, because he advocated a different, less expensive, hemostatic drug at The Cleveland Clinic. I would have greatly enjoyed conversing more with this great surgeon, but I was required to take a formal leave after 30 minutes.

The next session was with Ronald Elkins from Oklahoma, who presented an elderly patient who required a coronary artery bypass operation and a younger patient who had sustained a major blunt trauma to the chest. The third questioner was Peter Pairolero from the Mayo

Clinic, who presented a patient with postoperative pleural space problems and another patient with esophageal cancer. The final questioner was Frederick Grover, who presented a patient with adult respiratory distress syndrome and another with a left hilar mass. Overall, the examination went well, with the exception of my performance in the room of Ronald Elkins, where it seemed that whatever I said provoked a negative response.

After the examination, I had an enjoyable lunch with Benjamin Sun, a former general surgical trainee at UNC who had completed his cardiothoracic training at Columbia University. After a year on the faculty at Columbia, he had just accepted a job at Pennsylvania State University in Hershey. His primary interest was mechanical cardiac support systems, which was emphasized during his training at Columbia. He insisted on paying for lunch, because he was already an "attending" and I was still a "resident."

Much of Friday night before the examination I spent with with James Zellner, my friend who was an Assistant Professor of Surgery at the Medical University of South Carolina. He was extremely well prepared for the examination, as usual, but Delta Airlines had lost his luggage! Consequently, he had no suit to wear for his 10 a.m. examination on Saturday. I asked him what he intended to do, and he said that he would call Dr. Fred A. Crawford, Jr., his chairman at South Carolina, early in the morning to inform him and ask his advice. He predicted that Crawford's response would be, "Jim, this is poor planning on your part." When Zellner appeared at 10 a.m., as I exited my examination, he was wearing the concierge's dark suit and his own tennis shoes. Despite his appearance, he passed the test!

I also saw old friends from days at the National Institutes of Health: Patrick Griffith and his wife Petrinella, who lived in Ohio; and Jamie Holland, who was also in private practice in Ohio. On Friday during the day, I walked across Michigan Avenue to Brooks Brothers and bought two suits. The first was a light blue seersucker, which I had always wanted in the hot climate of North Carolina; and the second was a dark blue light-weight suit, which also seemed suitable for the summer.

On Saturday afternoon, I left Chicago for Dallas. My father greeted me at the airport and we returned to his home. We dressed and then dined at the Highland Park Cafe, one of his favorite restaurants. The staff greeted him on a first-name basis and treated us to complimentary hors d'ouevres and, after dinner, a glass of port. On Sunday, we retrieved from his office all the medical drawings of Leon Schlosberg from his 30 years at NIH. While my father was at work on Monday, I organized the drawings into separate categories and prepared them for storage. They are undoubtedly prized possessions that will adorn the walls of a medical library or conference room somewhere in the future.

My father imparted his usual wisdom during the trip. He gave me some particular financial advice, which was useful. He said that being debt-free was the key to life, and never to have a credit card debt. I listened to this complacently, because having been in cardiac surgical training for 11 years, I had known no other state than debt. He was recently married to Carrita Smith, who was still in Washington at the time of my visit to Dallas. She was sending much of her furniture to Dallas, and my father offered to give me a good deal of his. This was music to my ears, because I had only a dresser and some file cabinets in storage in Chapel Hill. We arranged for the movers to get the furniture and keep it in storage for six weeks until I had purchased a home in Chapel Hill.

On Tuesday, I flew to Chapel Hill for the specific purpose of buying a home. I had arranged to spend Wednesday morning with Ralph Pickett, a surgical assistant who is a part-time real estate agent. Because I had been with Lydia in search of a home in the Chapel Hill area on multiple occasions, I focused on two particular subdivisions. I had rented a car, and on Tuesday night drove to one of the subdivisions of interest, which was a group of townhouses off Airport Road, about five minutes from downtown Chapel Hill. The subdivision sat up on a hill, which was appealing; but when I walked around one of the new townhouses about 7 p.m., I could hear the roar of traffic down the hill.

From then on, I looked only at Southern Village, a new community situated about five minutes by car from the hospital. The agent at Southern Village awaited Pickett and me on Wednesday morning and took us to several homes. Fortunately, the first home she took us to interested me. A Charleston-style home sitting upon a hill, it had a good view of the surrounding woods. There were three bedrooms, a two-car garage, and porches on the ground floor level and the second level. After looking at several other homes that morning, I called Lydia in London, who had just returned from Paris, and we decided upon that first home, on Overlake Drive.

I met with Dr. Wilcox briefly on Wednesday and gave him a copy of *Memoirs of an Infantry Officer,* by Siegfried Sassoon, having read and thoroughly enjoyed a different copy of the book earlier in the year.

On Thursday morning, I flew to Nashville to visit Amelia and Camille. The anticipation of seeing them after being apart so long would rise for weeks. After arriving, I waited for my mother, Carey Roberts, to arrive from Washington, D.C., then we picked up the girls that afternoon.

As always, we met running with outstretched arms. It was a delightful four days, which we spent at AmeriSuites in Brentwood, just outside of Nashville. The weather was good, for the most part, and so we swam almost every day in the outdoor swimming pool, which the girls and I loved to do together. Their reading was improving, and they told me all about their teachers and friends. As usual, Camille asked to be carried when she got tired, and then Amelia requested her turn, out of fairness. Amelia, in her gentle way, observed people constantly, sometimes at point-blank range, and Camille, in her expressive way, was busy with her drawings and letters.

One evening we went to the Wild Horse Saloon on Second Avenue in downtown Nashville, and the girls took line dancing lessons while Mother and I dined. The highlight of the trip, however, was on Saturday, when we went to a remote farm outside of Nashville and enjoyed a long trail ride on horses. Each girl rode independently and managed well. One day we went to the Science Museum in Nashville, and the exhibit on the organ systems of the human body was particularly impressive. Several prominent physicians and surgeons at Vanderbilt University had donated money to create this exhibit.

We also made our usual visit to the Davis-Kidd Bookstore, where I bought Amelia and Camille some books. My mother bought me two books for my birthday, one called *Machine Art and Other Writings: The Lost Thought of the Italian Years,* by Ezra Pound, which I read on the airplane coming home, and the other was *The Complete Correspondence Between Thomas Jefferson and Abigail and John Adams,* edited by Lester J. Capone, which I read during my last month in London. On Sunday, I parted from my mother and Amelia and Camille, which was never easy, and returned to London by way of Raleigh, North Carolina.

In general terms, the 10-day trip was a success. I had passed the oral examination by the American Board of Thoracic Surgery, had a wonderful visit with my father and arranged to purchase and furnish a home in Chapel Hill, and finally, had a splendid visit with my darling daughters and mother. In London on Monday morning, June 16, I reunited with Lydia at 21 St. Luke's Street. The jet lag was always more difficult to bear when going from the States to London.

I made three trips home during the year in London and always returned with some small gift for Lincoln, usually some uniquely American food or drink. I brought barbecue sauce from both eastern and western North Carolina, there being a great difference in the taste, some preserves from Tennessee, Makers Mark bourbon, maple syrup from Vermont, etc.—things American.

Chapter 26

Stoking the Fire

The book of surgery I took to London by Kirklin and Barratt-Boyes I read regularly throughout the year. My surgical education in London, however, occurred primarily in the operating theater. During the one-year period (August 1, 1996, to July 31, 1997), Lincoln performed or supervised 352 operations on NHS patients and performed an additional 124 operations on private patients at the RBH, the Wellington Hospital, or the Harley Street Clinic.

I cannot report that the sailing was smooth the entire year. I arrived in London thinking that I was fully prepared, when, in fact, I had a lot to learn. The biggest initial challenge was getting comfortable again in the operating theater. After an exhausting year as chief resident in cardiac surgery at UNC, I took off the month of July—one entire month with no operating; really, no medical reading at all. When I arrived at the RBH in August, I was physically fit and ready, but suddenly mentally insecure about operating, having been away from it for a month. One month would not matter, had I already been operating *independently* in cardiac surgery.

Another problem was that many instruments and techniques used by Lincoln were new to me. I learned one or two ways to do things at UNC. Now I was confronted with a third way. The electrocautery device, for example, was a sort of pencil with a tip, and one operated it in the States by pushing a button on the pencil with a finger. At the RBH, I was handed an electrocautery stick with a *foot* pedal. This seemingly simple difference caused me great anxiety at first—like suddenly driving a stick shift automobile, after driving an automatic for 10 years.

After cannulating the aorta for cardiopulmonary bypass in some 400 patients at UNC, I asked for the same small dilator I had used routinely and was given a side-biting clamp instead, which was Lincoln's method of cannulating. I struggled briefly with that. I asked for a pair of fine dissecting scissors one day to expose a coronary artery in epicardial fat and was handed only a scalpel. The round needle holder I was handed kept slipping out of my green-gloved hands until I realized that the alternative white gloves were not slippery. I made one ungraceful move after another, all under the watchful eye of Lincoln, in the first three months. I began to question whether I was worthy of his attention.

I was sent from the surgeon's side of the table to the assistant's side a couple of times. Lincoln would say to someone watching this spectacle, "Charles is in the doghouse." I was unaccustomed to his method of teaching. When I operated at first, he did not scrub in, but rather watched from behind the ether screen. But I must say, after sending me to the assistant's side of the table, he would turn over the next case to me. For example, I began a mitral valve replacement which he took over, but the next case he let me do, a coarctation repair in a child.

At one point in the first three months, I asked a nurse if what I was experiencing was in any way unusual for a trainee under Lincoln. This kind Chinese nurse told me that I was doing okay as long as Lincoln did not kick me out of the room. She told me that he had in the past told trainees to leave the operating theater and not return until he said so. One man he sent to the ICU with instructions to stay there and look after patients until he indicated otherwise. Another man he sent to his office to perform the duties of his secretary for two weeks while she was away on holiday. Another man, now a prominent pediatric cardiac surgeon in London, he commanded to stand in the corner of the operating theater and face the wall. Lincoln was known to say, "How can I soar with the eagles when I am surrounded by turkeys," which fortunately, I never heard.

For the first five months I assisted Lincoln, only very rarely operating independently, apart from opening and closing the chest. Around Christmas, however, he said, "You have seen how I do the operations, Charles. In the new year, you will do them." Indeed, the last seven months were extremely enjoyable. Certain pediatric operations—repair of an atrial septal defect, coarctation of the aorta, and patent ductus arteriosus—Lincoln routinely turned over to me or the senior registrar, Tony Desouza, and Lincoln did not scrub in to assist. Toward the end of the operation, he would usually appear at the door in his suit, leaning in. "Is everything all right, Charles?" "Yes, sir." "Thank you," and he would disappear.

In most of the pediatric cardiac operations, however, I still assisted Lincoln, but he let me do more—cannulate, wean from cardiopulmonary bypass, and decannulate. He also routinely let me open the chest in children who had had previous cardiac operations. Scarring in the chest makes these reoperations more difficult than a first-time operation. I occasionally did the adult operations, as well, such as coronary artery bypass or aortic valve replacement.

Some weeks were busier than others. During the week of Sunday, May 4, 1997, for example, Lincoln performed or supervised fifteen operations at the RBH, three of which were on private patients. Assisted by Tony Desouza and Jeremy Prout, I performed repair of an aortic coarctation in a two-day-old child, coronary bypass in a 53-year-old man, coronary bypass in a 75-year-old man, closure of an atrial septal defect in a 33-year-old woman, and closure of a patent ductus arteriosus in a three-year-old girl. Lincoln assisted me in the closure of a ventricular septal defect in a three-month-old boy. I assisted Lincoln in three operations: repair of an aortic coarctation in a five-month-old boy, pulmonary arterial banding and closure of a patent ductus arteriosus in a two-month-old girl, and an aortic valve replacement in an 80-year-old woman. Desouza assisted Lincoln in relieving right ventricular outflow obstruction after an arterial switch in a three-year-old boy. I assisted Desouza on a minimally invasive coronary bypass in a 64-year-old man and the closure of a patent ductus arteriosus in a seven-month-old girl. That was a busy week. I participated in exactly 300 operations during the year, about 25 a month.

What I learned from Lincoln was the importance of keeping cardiac operations simple. He did not add unnecessary maneuvers that distract attention and prolong the procedure. He believed that "every unnecessary extra minute in theater results in ten minutes additional time in the ICU." His pediatric cardiac surgical results, in particular, were superb because the infant or child got a well-planned, efficient operation. That Lincoln placed sutures well, cut patches well to close holes in the heart, dissected carefully—this goes without saying.

The coronary bypass operation was the most common operation he performed or that was performed under his supervision, and his methods were safe and simple. He rarely did combined procedures, such as carotid endarterectomy in the setting of coronary bypass. He never did sequential graft anastomoses, and he never gave retrograde cardioplegia. His myocardial preservation technique was uniform—cold crystalloid cardioplegia delivered in antegrade fashion with ice slush applied topically. He usually did two distal anastomoses before repeating a half dose of cardioplegia. He did not vent the heart, only the aortic root through the cardioplegia cannula, and did not place pacing wires. "I do not use pacing wires," he said, "in conventional heart operations for conventional heart diseases." When I first-assisted him in a coronary bypass, he said, "The only thing to observe in this operation is how I make the proximal anastomosis." He used a scalpel, not a punch, to make the hole in the aorta, and the vein graft he opened rather long, so that the vein was fixed to the aorta like a cobra head.

For heart valve operations, he had several rules, which he emphasized by saying, "I want these words tatooed on my chest: 'Use no continuous suture in the heart,' or 'Use only a Starr-Edwards valve,' or 'Close my aortotomy in two layers.'"

What I also observed about Lincoln was how to conduct a busy practice of cardiac surgery—when to operate, when not to operate, when to come in, when to go home, when to call, when to consult others, etc. Lincoln conserved his energy for the operation—the planning of it and the execution of it. When the operation was done with, he was able to go home, usually by 7 p.m. The senior registrars typically looked after the patients overnight. He would always call, but he had to rest for the next day. This was how he maintained stamina in a consultant practice of 23 years.

In this world of beepers and portable telephones, Lincoln had neither. But strangely, he was never unreachable when I needed to talk to him, except once. He had performed a pericardiectomy on a private patient at the RBH, and the patient was having a stormy postoperative course. At one point, an attempt was made to withdraw a central venous catheter from his left jugular vein. The catheter would not budge, as it had been inadvertently sewn into a vein in the mediastinum (middle of the chest). Unable to reach Lincoln, I took the patient back to the operating theater, reopened his chest, found the culprit stitch and cut it, freeing the catheter inside the vein. This was the only time during the year I needed to speak with Lincoln and he was inaccessible. Of course he called late that evening, was informed of the events, and received the information unperturbed.

It must be said that his surgical career dominated his life. He gave his energy overwhelmingly to it, at the expense of other interests. He did not watch television, and he saw a movie for the first time in 20 years when I was there. He took life from patient to patient, operation to operation, and achieved a level of excellence that few in the profession reach. If my child was born with a congenital defect of the heart, he or she would fare no better than under the care of Lincoln.

Chapter 27

Former Trainees of Lincoln

Lincoln recalled many anecdotes related to his former trainees. He took pride when his trainees landed in good institutions in the UK and abroad, remarking once that he "trained everyone at Oxford," more recently including Stephen Westaby, Ravi Pillai, and David Taggart. Pillai was at Lincoln's Christmas party in December. Lincoln was also proud of the new consultant surgeon at Great Ormond Street, Victor Tsang, a former trainee, whose first consultant post was at Southhampton. Tsang replaced the Czech, Jarda Stark, who retired in December 1996.

Lincoln spoke occasionally of his previous American fellows, Kirk Kantor, who is now a pediatric cardiac surgeon at Emory University, and Sara Shumway, a cardiothoracic surgeon at the University of Minnesota. About Shumway, he remarked, "Tim Gardner called me from Hopkins and asked me if I would train a woman. I said, 'I don't really want a girl.' He said, 'Before you answer, let me tell you her last name: Shumway.'" Sara Shumway's father was the renowned cardiac surgeon at Stanford University, Norman Shumway, a pioneer in heart transplantation.

Lincoln had visited Stanford briefly and had great admiration for Norman Shumway. He liked to repeat a comment Shumway made to one of his trainees during an operation. While a trainee at Stanford paused momentarily at the operating table, Shumway said, "Keep working. You can always do *something* toward completing the operation." Lincoln operated with this principle, as well. When the cardiac portion of the operation was completed, he rarely paused. While the patient was rewarming on the heart-lung machine, he would put the chest drains in, stop any minor bleeding, etc. Lincoln liked Shumway's self-description as "the greatest first assistant in the world."

About Sara Shumway, he remarked, “We tried to get her to say ‘bloody‘ correctly, but at the end of the year she still did not get it right. She had a sense of humor, like her father.” About another American trainee he once remarked, “He is a fine surgeon, but he has the most boring personality I have ever known in the world.” Lincoln once commented, “My worst fellow was an American. I could not teach him anything, but I did learn one thing from him. He was taught in America to size the aortic valve during an aortic valve replacement, then select one size smaller.”

Lincoln trained surgeons differently than American educators. With Lincoln’s method, one watched or assisted him and then, when ready, did the operation independently, assisted by a junior trainee. Lincoln himself rarely first-assisted, except in some pediatric cardiac operations. If Lincoln came into the room when one of his trainees was operating as surgeon, he would not infrequently carry on conversations with the anesthetist, the nurse, or the surgeon himself. I found this to be somewhat distracting and tried to ignore it, unless he was addressing me directly.

He disliked slow surgery, and I remember assisting a registrar in the fall who came into Lincoln’s view from above the ether screen. “Move along. If you want to think, you should do neurosurgery . . . or psychiatry.” He told one assistant, “You need to think faster, boy”—and to another slow assistant in the middle of the operation, he said, “Imagine you are here.”

During the year, Lincoln was asked to offer an opinion in a medicolegal case involving one of his former American trainees in Arizona. The American surgeon’s defense attorneys sought Lincoln’s advice concerning a child who had sustained brain injury during a rare operation that Lincoln had performed several times. Lincoln came into the registrar’s office where I was seated one day and asked to borrow my copy of the book by Kirklin and Barratt-Boyes. He sat down several desks away and looked up the section on the bidirectional Glenn operation to find out what was said about brain injury.

The case involved a child who had undergone a bidirectional Glenn operation *without* using cardiopulmonary bypass. An expert witness on the plaintiff’s side had claimed that it was unacceptable to perform that operation without cardiopulmonary bypass. Over his 23-year consultant career, however, Lincoln had performed the operation about half a dozen times through a right thoracotomy *without* cardiopulmonary bypass.

The operation was, of course, rare, but Lincoln had had no major complications. About that particular operation, he once remarked that it was the only time his hand shook while sewing. During the year, Lincoln performed the operation twice, and it was indeed the only time I ever saw his hand shake. After he completed the second operation, he said to me, "Charles, you will not tell Wilcox about this, will you?"

Lincoln came in one morning and said, "Your predecessor did his first switch" (arterial switch operation for transposition of the great arteries). My predecessor was, of course, the son of Professor Carlos Moraes from Recife, Brazil. He gave the Brazilian fellow a new round-handled needle-holder as a parting gift.

Lincoln also mentioned a previous trainee named Julian Gaer, who went on to work with Carpentier in Paris before recently obtaining a consultant position at St. George's Hospital. Lincoln related a story about Gaer at an early stage in his training: "I told him to quit cardiac surgery. . . . Gaer called me that night to say that he had considered my advice, but was not going to take it." Gaer spoke fluent French, Lincoln said, and it was therefore easier for him to secure a position with Carpentier. Later in his training, Gaer apparently told Lincoln that Carpentier did not write a recommendation for him when he applied for the consultant position at St. George's Hospital, the reason being that "the French do not understand how to do it." Perhaps they do not fill the letters with glowing words and exaggerated praises, as we tend to do in the States.

He also related the story of one previous trainee who had done a mitral valve replacement independently under his "supervision" in the middle of the night. Lincoln was not present during the operation and assumed that the trainee had used interrupted sutures to secure the valve in the annulus, which was Lincoln's usual technique that he insisted that everyone do while on his service. The patient returned to the hospital a month or so later in acute congestive heart failure. Lincoln did not suspect dehiscence of the suture line because he had assumed that interrupted sutures had been placed. Nevertheless, Lincoln reoperated on the patient on a Saturday night, which of course he hated to do. At operation, they found almost complete dehiscence (separation) of the mitral valve prosthesis from the annulus. It was apparent that a continuous suture line had been used. Lincoln was furious and described the incident to me as a "breach of trust." The senior registrar who had performed the operation told Lincoln that he had been in a hurry and the nurses were not efficient; that is why he had used continuous rather than interrupted sutures, which take longer.

Though Lincoln might appear to some to be arrogant, he was, in fact, quite humble about his own difficulties in the practice of surgery. He told me time and time again about his repeated failure to pass the Royal College of Surgeons exam, early in his training. "It ruined your life. You would be at a pub with a girl thinking that you should be studying." Lincoln could master certain parts of the exam at certain times, he said, but not all parts at one time. "I could not keep it all in my head."

He described his fourth or fifth sitting for the examination, when he was presented with a patient with a neck mass. Lincoln proceeded to list several possible diagnoses, and then he said, "I know it is not malignant." The examiner asked, "How do you know it is not malignant?" Lincoln replied, "Because this man was presented to me in this exam two years ago."

Sometime after he finally passed, Lincoln awakened one night from sleep and could not convince himself that he had indeed passed the examination. He thought he had only dreamed it. He rose from bed, dressed, and drove to the old Brompton. The porter at the door asked, "Mr. Lincoln, why have you come? No one has called you." Lincoln replied that he came to see a patient. Instead, he went to his file cabinet and found the document stating that he was indeed a Fellow of the Royal College of Surgeons.

When a junior surgeon was working on the leg or groin, Lincoln once said, "I never could close the groin vessels. Someone always had to come down to help me." Humble remarks like this, of course, make a trainee feel less incapable in the presence of a formidable cardiac surgeon. "I didn't understand most of what I was doing as an SHO (senior house officer)," he remarked once at the operating table. To me he would occasionally say, "Charles, you have wasted the year. You should have worked for de Leval."

At the operating table during the year, Lincoln told me of surgical errors he had made in his 23 years in practice. I had never heard an American surgeon speak so candidly of their own errors. Usually, surgeons refrain from discussing their complications, particularly fatal ones. Lincoln told me candidly of specific mistakes he had made over the years, and this frankness did not diminish his stature, but indeed, increased it. Of fatal errors, he said, "You will take them with you to the grave."

While operating with trainees, it was Lincoln's habit to offer regular breaks to his assistants during a long operation. Only two or three times in ten years in the States had anyone offered me a break from assisting at a long operation. With Lincoln, it was routine. As soon as we finished the important technical part of the procedure and had begun rewarming on cardiopulmonary bypass, Lincoln would say, "Charles, go have a cup of coffee." When I returned, he would often scrub out of the operation and have a cup of tea, sometimes returning to the table only to supervise from above the ether screen. He told me jokingly that Haznat Khan, his former registrar, would go to the roof of the RBH to smoke cigarettes and not return for 30 minutes!

Lincoln had many visitors to his operating theater from various countries. Norwegian surgeons appeared one day; a Nigerian surgeon, Martin A.C.Aghaji, stayed for a few days; a Czech surgeon came; an Argentine came; even an American medical student appeared one day. In general, Lincoln liked to debrief people, both visitors to the RBH and the RBH trainees who went away and came back.

Rajiv Chaturvedi was a senior registrar in pediatric cardiology at the RBH who took a job on the faculty at Boston Children's Hospital in January 1997. During the year, Chaturvedi had carried on a study on left ventricular function on patients of Lincoln in the operating theater. Despite the occasional inconvenience involved in inserting pressure catheters, and taking measurements at the end of the operation, Lincoln was quite willing to participate in the study, which was later published (Chaturvedi RR, Lincoln C, Gothard JWW, et al: *J Thorac Cardiovasc Surg* 1998;115:77–83).

When Chaturvedi returned to London to visit in the spring, he brought Lincoln a Harvard tie. Lincoln called me into his office while he was debriefing Chateverdi on protocols at the Boston Children's Hospital. Lincoln was always interested in how surgery was practiced elsewhere. I do not mean to suggest that he would casually change his own methods. He would not. But he was curious and would adopt a new technique or practice if it was sensible. He was particularly interested in improving the postoperative care of the children. He was never entirely satisfied with the pediatric ICU at the RBH.

Whenever a member of his team went to a surgical meeting, Lincoln called a small team conference to allow the trainee to share the information and experience. Tony Desouza became interested in performing coronary bypasses without the heart-lung machine, for example, a relatively new idea in cardiac surgery. Lincoln sent him to meetings, had him present his findings, and then allowed Tony to carry out the operations under his supervision. I found this progressive thinking quite admirable, particularly for a senior surgeon near the end of his career.

Lincoln had a separate fund from which he drew to pay for meetings for his trainees. "If I don't spend it, it will go to my colleagues," he would say. During the year he paid for me to attend meetings at Liverpool, Harefield Hospital, Prague, the RBH, and Dublin. As I mentioned earlier, he gave me a book by Hurt on *The History of Cardiothoracic Surgery,* and he would deposit in my mailbox during the year articles on various subjects ranging from cuff links to congenital heart defects.

Chapter 28

The Wedding and Departure

Upon my return from the States in June, Lydia and I decided to marry while in London. She made arrangements at the Chelsea Town Hall, which was one block from our home, to marry on Friday, July 11. Although it was a small ceremony, it was nevertheless very enjoyable and romantic. Lydia's younger brother, David Warren, was my best man, and Lydia's maid of honor was Leslie Jeng.

The preceding Wednesday night I was on call at the hospital and did not sleep at home. On Thursday night, it was decided that I would sleep at the flat of Francis Ferdinand and that Leslie would stay with Lydia at our flat on St. Luke's Street. When Lydia appeared that Friday morning, she looked stunning in her white dress and large English hat. Photographs were taken on the steps of the Chelsea Town Hall after the brief ceremony. Cyrus and Judy Wilson, our American friends, hosted a delightful brunch of champagne, orange juice, quiche, and pastries at their home on Park Walk. Francis and Leslie attended the ceremony, as did Tony Desouza, Lorraine Spencer, and her three children. Leslie Valente, a nurse from Chicago and friend of Leslie and Lydia working temporarily at the RBH, also came.

After brunch, Lydia and I took a taxi to the Ritz on Picadilly Road to spend the night. A bottle of champagne awaited us in the room, along with fruit and peanuts, and a beautiful view of Green Park from the balcony. That evening, we celebrated our wedding at Ostreria la Fate, an Italian restaurant in Chelsea. Our party was accommodated in a candlelit room with wine bottles on shelves covering the walls. Cyrus and Judy Wilson, Francis and Leslie, and Tony and Sarah, as well as Lydia's brother David, came. Sarah had a couple visiting her, and they came, as well. After dinner, Lydia and I retired to the Ritz and had a "lie in" (sleeping in late), as they say in London, on Saturday morning. At 11 a.m., we enjoyed an English breakfast in the Ritz dining room before returning home to St. Luke's Street.

That afternoon, I took David, Lydia's brother, to the Imperial War Museum south of the Thames. I had intended all year to go there. It was an extraordinary museum, with particularly good exhibits on the World Wars. While the loss of life as a consequence of World War I was about 15,000,000, the loss of life in World World II was about 50,000,000, according to the museum figures.

That evening, Tony and Sarah Desouza hosted a cookout to celebrate our wedding. Francis and Leslie joined us, along with David Warren and Leslie Valente. On the grounds beside the Thames with a portable barbecue, Desouza cooked four meats: beefsteak, chicken, lamb, and sausage. We brought it all upstairs and had a feast in his living room. Somehow we found room for dessert, and then we relaxed to good music, while Ferdinand slept and Desouza sang.

Lydia arranged to fly into Charlotte on Tuesday, July 24, and I had a return ticket to Atlanta on Thursday, July 26. During the last week, we packed our bags, trying to limit ourselves to three pieces of luggage each. We gave away some of our meager possessions: a lamp to Cyrus and Judy Wilson, our iron and several dishes to Leslie and Francis, etc. On Friday night, July 20, Lydia and I were invited to Cyrus and Judy Wilson's home for dinner. I had enjoyed their company over the year so very much, it was hard to imagine that we would soon be an ocean apart. They gave us a lovely wedding gift: an antique knife and fork set.

The following night, Lydia and I went to the home of Lincoln and Karen Jurgens for a farewell dinner. Two weeks before, Karen had asked me to make a list of people whom I would like to invite to this dinner. On this list I included Francis Ferdinand and Leslie Jeng, Tony Desouza and his wife Sarah, Melanie Cheung and her fiancé Andrew Cohen, Jeremy Prout, the senior house officer on Lincoln's service, and his girlfriend, Vincent Young and his wife, and Cyrus and Judy Wilson.

The Wilsons took us to Pembroke Square in their brand-new green Volvo, and Lincoln and Karen came outside to greet us. It was the first time that either Karen or Lincoln had met Lydia or the Wilsons, about whom I had spoken many times before. We had champagne in the garden before dinner.

Lincoln gathered everyone around at one point and made a presentation to me of a couple of gifts. The first was a "Roberts clamp," which is similar to a tonsil or Burlisher clamp at UNC. He told the story of how he would ask for this surgical instrument during an operation by saying

"Roberts" and I would respond unwittingly, "Yes, sir." Of course I soon realized that he was asking for the instrument, but it made an amusing story. He then described me as "the best dressed man at the Brompton Hospital," which of course was untrue, and presented me with two blue cuff links. Jeremy Prout, the senior house officer, gave me a polka-dotted blue tie from Thomas Pink on Jermyn Street, and Melanie gave me a book of photographs of Chelsea. Earlier in the evening, Lydia brought Karen some flowers, and I gave Lincoln two books. One was a new account of the British aviators in World War I, and the other was a complete edition of Boswell's biography of Samuel Johnson.

The food that evening was sumptuous. I was told, though I cannot confirm it, that Lincoln cooked the main courses and Karen prepared the two delicious desserts. There was a roast beef, numerous baked quails, and a seafood and rice dish that was delicious. Lincoln prepared the chutney, and there were several fruits and vegetables to complement the main courses. We took our plates into the candlelit garden, where we sat at antique tables and chairs. Lincoln and Karen moved in and out of the garden, keeping everyone's wine glass full and encouraging us to go back for seconds.

It could not have been a more pleasant evening. Lydia told me later that Lincoln took her hand and said that when he was in Alabama, he had seen what is meant by the "Southern belle." He said that he believed in that concept and that she was, indeed, a Southern belle. Judy Wilson told me the next day that she had a wonderful time, marveling at how effortlessly Lincoln and Karen seemed to carry off this splendid dinner party in their garden. Lincoln took Cyrus Wilson into the house at one point and showed him the privately bound book of letters of his great-uncle, the young aviator who was killed in The Great War.

What I learned in London will be measured best by how well my patients fare in subsequent years, I suppose, but some learning experiences are unquantifiable. It is regrettable that not every surgeon-in-training comes within the sphere of a great teacher like Mr. Christopher Lincoln. Part of the purpose of this book was to describe the sphere in which I trained for a year. On my last day at the RBH, I reopened a child's chest and then assisted Lincoln on yet another complicated re-operation. When the difficult part was finally completed, he held out his hand across the operating table in silence, and I shook it. He walked away from the patient, and I went from the assistant's side to the surgeon's side, where I have remained.

Appendix I

Christopher Lincoln: Bibliography

Journal Articles

1. Lincoln JCR. Cervico-auricular fistulae. Arch Dis Children 1965;40:210.
2. Lincoln JCR. Leiomyosarcoma of the anterior mediastinum. Thorax 1965;20:362.
3. Lincoln JCR. Malignant argentaffinoma with metastases to the ovaries. Br J Surg 1966;53:1071.
4. Lightman DJ, Lincoln JCR. Malignant pulmonary interstitial emphysema. Br J Anaes 1967;39:587.
5. Lincoln JCR, Tynan MJ, Waterston DJ. Successful excision of an endocardial fibroma of the left ventricle in a ten month old infant. J Thor Cardiovasc Surg 1968;56:63.
6. Lincoln JCR, Stark J, Tynan MJ, Aberdeen E. Constriction (banding) of Blalock-Taussig anastomosis for intractable congestive cardiac failure and pulmonary oedema. Thorax 1968;23:524.
7. Deverall PB, Lincoln JCR, Aberdeen E, Bonham-Carter RE, Waterston DJ. Surgical management of triicuspid atresia. Thorax 1969;24:239.
8. Deverall PB, Aberdeen E, Bonham-Carter RE, Waterston DJ, Lincoln JCR. Aortopulmonary window. J Thorac Cardiovasc Surg 1969;57:479.
9. Lincoln JCR, Deverall PB, Stark J, Aberdeen E, Waterston DJ. Vascular anomalies compressing the oesophagus and trachea. Thorax 1969;24:295.
10. Lincoln JCR, Deverall PB. The treatment of arterial thrombosis in infants and children by balloon catheters. J Paediatr Surg 1969;4:359.
11. Lincoln JCR, Barnes ND, Gould T, Reynolds EOR. Pulmonary mechanics and surfactant measurement in canine lungs following reimplantation. Thorax 1970;25(2):180.
12. Kazemi H, Bruecke P, Parsons EF, Lincoln JCR. Hypoxic pulmonary vascular response: Role of the autonomic nervous system. Fed Proc Atlantic City 1970;29:270.
13. Lincoln JCR, Valenca LM, Kazemi H, Austen WG. Serial perfusion and ventilation studies following reimplantation of the lung using xenon 133, pulmonary angiography and bronchography. J Thorac Cardiovasc Surg 1970;60:108.
14. Lincoln JCR, Proven JL. Mediastinoscopy in the diagnosis of non-malignant thoracic disease. J Thorac Cardiovasc Surg 1970;60:144.

15. Lowenstein E, Lincoln JCR, Modell JH, Austen WG, Laver MB. Preservation of excised canine lungs by ventilation with liquid fluorocarbon. Fed Proc (Atlantic City) 1970;29:1775.
16. Lincoln JCR, Lowenstein E, Austen WG, Laver MB. Acute effects of autotransplantation on pulmonary vascular resistance and blood-gas exchange in the canine lung. Ann Surg 1970;172:877 (also Br J Surg 1970; 57:852).
17. Balcon R, Emanuel R, Lincoln JCR, McDonald L, Ross D, Somerville J. Fascia lata replacement of isolated aortic valve disease: A followup of 23 cases from the National Heart Hospital, London. CV Res VI World Congr Cardiol 1970;70.
18. Lincoln JCR, Balcon R, Emanuel R, McDonald L, Muir J, Ross DN, Somerville J, Taylor J. Mitral valve replacement with fascia lata. CV Res VI World Congr Cardiol 1970;200.
19. Lincoln JCR, Stark J, Subramanian S, Aberdeen E, Bonham-Carter RE, Berry CL, Waterston DJ. Congenital lobar emphysema. Ann Surg 1971; 173:55.
20. Schottenfeld M, Wisheart JD, Ross JK, Lincoln JCR, Ross DN. Cloth destruction and haemolysis with totally cloth-covered Starr-Edwards prostheses. Thorax 1971;26:159.
21. Lincoln C, Geens M, Ross D, Ionescu M. Replacement of pulmonary valve and pulmonary artery with fascia lata. Br Heart J 1971;33:146.
22. Lincoln JCR, Riley PA, Revignas A, Geens M, Ross DN, Ross JK. The viability of autologous fascia lata in heart valve replacements. Thorax 1971;26:277.
23. Valenca LM, Lincoln JCR, Strieder DJ, Kazemi H. Pulmonary vascular response of the reimplanted dog lung to hypoxia. J Thorac Cardiovasc Surg 1971;61:857.
24. Lincoln JCR, Geens M, Schottenfeld M, Ross DN. Pulmonary valve replacement with fascia lata. Ann Thorac Surg 1972;13:104.
25. Lincoln JCR. Total correction of D-loop double outlet right ventricle with bilateral conus, L-transposition and pulmonic stenosis. J Thorac Cardiovasc Surg 1972;64:435.
26. Lincoln JCR. The early, intermediate, and late function of the auto-transplanted lung. Ann Roy Coll Surg Eng 1972;51:299.
27. Ross JK, Lincoln JCR, Sapsford RN, Wisheart J. Natural history of fascia lata valves in the aortic and mitral positions. Thorax 1973;28:458.
28. Reid KG, Lincoln JCR. Successful repair of acute traumatic left subclavian artery steal syndrome. Proc Roy Soc Med 1973;66:911.
29. Manenti A, Lincoln JCR. Extrapleural haemothorax from rupture of the subclavian artery. Gazzetts Sanitaria 1973;22:120.

30. Rees A, Symons J, Joseph MC, Lincoln JCR. Ventricular septal defect in a battered child. Br Med J 1975;1:20.
31. Lincoln JCR, Anderson RH, Shinebourne EA, English TAH, Wilkinson JL. Double outlet right ventricle with L-malposition of the aorta. Br Heart J 1975;37:453.
32. Paneth M, Lennox SC, Lincoln JCR, Joseph MC, Shinebourne EA. [Critical outflow valve obstruction under the age of one year (author's translation)]. [German] Thoraxchir Vaskulare Chirurgie 1975;23:459.
33. Lennox SC, Lincoln JCR, Paneth M, Shinebourne EA, Joseph MC. Critical outflow valve obstruction under the age of one year. Br Heart J 1975; 37:554.
34. Wyse SD, Pfitzner J, Rees A, Lincoln JCR, Branthwaite MA. Measurement of cardiac output by thermal dilution in infants and children. Thorax 1975;30:262.
35. Hasse J, Lincoln JCR, Paneth M. Differentiated surgical therapy in congenital lobar emphysema (German). Thoraxchir Vaskulare Chirurgie 1975; 23:250.
36. Honey M, Lincoln JCR, Osborne MP, de Bono DP. Coarctation of aorta with right aortic arch. Br Heart J 1975;37:937.
37. Lincoln JCR. Totally corrective cardiac surgery in the first two years of life. Proc Royal Soc Med 1975;68:716.
38. Lincoln JCR, Shinebourne EA, Joseph MC, Gibson RV, Anderson RH. Surgical repair of conotruncal abnormalities. Br Heart J 1975;37:553.
39. Shinebourne EA, Tam ASY, Elseed AM, Paneth M, Lennox SC, Cleland WP, Lincoln JCR, Anderson RH. Coarctation of the aorta in infancy and childhood. Br Heart J 1976;38:375.
40. Armstrong RF, Southorn PA, Secker-Walker J, Lincoln JCR, Soutter L. Continuous monitoring of mixed venous oxygen tension. Br Med J 1976; 2:282.
41. Lincoln JCR, Hasse J, Anderson RH, Shinebourne EA. Surgical correction in complete laevotransposition of the great arteries with an unusual ventricular septal defect. Am J Cardiol 1976;38:44.
42. Armstrong RF, Hutchinson JM, Lincoln JCR, Ingram D, Soutter L. Continuous measurement of arterial oxygen tension during one-lung anaesthesia. Br J Anaesth 1976;48:1005.
43. Gibson D, Tse TF, Upton M, Lincoln JCR. Echocardiographic assessment of left ventricular filling in patients after Mustard's operation. Abstract book. European Cardiology Meeting, Amsterdam 1976.
44. Thompson DS, Westaby S, Lincoln JCR. Ventricular haemangioendothelioma diagnosed in life. Br Heart J 1977;39:462.
45. Lincoln JCR, Jamieson S, Joseph MC, Shinebourne EA, Anderson RH.

Transatrial repair of ventricular septal defect with reference to their anatomic classification. J Thorac Cardiovasc Sur 1977;74:183.
46. Jamieson SW, Lincoln JCR. Some effects of sulphinpyrazone in cardiac bypass surgery. Proceedings of a symposium organized by Geigy Pharmaceuticals, 1977.
47. Krayenbuhg CU, Lincoln JCR. Total anomalous systemic venous connection, common atrium and partial atrioventricular canal. J Thorac Cardiovasc Surg 1977;73:686.
48. Symons JC, Shinebourne EA, Joseph MC, Lincoln JCR, Ho Y, Anderson RH. Criss-cross heart with congenitally corrected transposition: A report of a case with D-transposed aorta and ventricular pre-excitation. Eur J Cardiol 1977;5:493.
49. Mustafa I, Shinebourne EA, Lincoln JCR. Successful replacement of the interventricular septum following excision of a large intramural fibroma. J Cardiovasc Surg 1978;19:411.
50. Wilkinson JL, Smith A, Lincoln JCR, Anderson RH. The conducting tissues in congenitally corrected transposition with situs inversus. Br Heart J 1978;40:41.
51. Armstrong RF, St. Andrew D, Cohen SL, Secker-Walker J, Cobbe SM, Lincoln JCR. Continuous monitoring of mixed venous oxygen tension (PV02) in cardiorespiratory disorders. Lancet 1978;1:632.
52. Lincoln JCR, Leanage R, Keeton B, Lam L Southall D, Shinebourne EA. A study of cardiac arrhythmias by ambulatory monitoring before and after Mustard's operation for transposition of the great arteries. Circulation 1978;11:148.
53. Lincoln JCR, McKay R, Miller GAH, Joseph MC, Shinebourne EA. Surgical correction of complete atrioventricular canal in infants and children. Br Heart J 1978;40:451.
54. Crupi GC, Anderson RH, Ho SY, Lincoln JCR. Complete transposition of the great arteries with intact ventricular septum and left ventricular outflow tract obstruction: Surgical management and anatomic considerations. J Thorac Cardiovasc Surg 1979;78:730.
55. Shinebourne EA, Southall DP, Keeton BR, Leanage R, Lam L, Lincoln JCR. Arrhythmias and Mustard's operation. Br Heart J 1979;41:367.
56. Lincoln JCR, Butler P, Logan-Sinclair R, Anderson RH. A cardiac conduction monitor and probe for intraoperative identification of conduction tissue. Br Heart J 1979;42:339.
57. Southall DP, Keeton BR, Leanage R, Lam L, Joseph MC, Anderson RH, Lincoln JCR, Shinebourne EA. Cardiac rhythm and conduction before and after Mustard's operation for complete transposition of the great arteries. Br Heart J 1980;43:21.

58. Lam LKT, Ward OC, Southall DP, Lincoln JCR. Mustard's operation for transposition of the great arteries: Surgical results and the incidence of cardiac arrhythmias. Irish Med J 1980;73:458.
59. Ullal RR, Anderson RH, Lincoln JCR. Mustard's operation modified to avoid dysrhythmias and pulmonary and systemic venous obstruction. J Thorac Cardiovasc Surg 1979;78:431.
60. Lincoln JCR, Treasure T. Some surgical considerations in complex congenital heart disease: Atrioventricular cana, tetralogy of Fallot, pulmonary atresia, simple and complex transposition of the great arteries. Indian Heart J; Teaching Series 1980;3:56.
61. Lau KC, Calcaterra G, Miller GAH, Lincoln JCR, Lennox SC, Paneth M, Anderson RH, Shinebourne EA. Aorto-pulmonary window. J Cardiovasc Surg 1982;23:21.
62. Crupi G, Anderson RH, Lincoln JCR. Complete transposition of the great arteries with intact ventricular septum and left ventricular outflow tract obstruction: Surgical management and anatomic considerations. J Thorac Cardiovasc Surg 1979;78:730.
63. Crupi G, Gibson D, Heard B, Lincoln JCR. Severe late failure of a porcine xenograft mitral valve: Clinical echocardiography and pathologic finding. Thorax 1980;35:210.
64. Gristwood RW, Lincoln JCR, Owen DAA. Effects of histamine on human isolated heart muscle: Comparison with effects of noradrenaline. J Pharm Pharmacol 1980;32:145.
65. Fisher C, Grubb C, Kenning B, Lincoln JCR. Pseudolymphoma of the lung: A rare cause of a solitary nodule. J Thorac Cardiovasc Surg 1980; 80:11.
66. Ross A, Lincoln JCR. Congenitally corrected transposition of the great arteries with tricuspid incompetence, successfully treated by xenograft valve replacement in a 15 month old child. Thorax 1981;36:217.
67. Gristwood RW, Lincoln JCR, Owen DAA, Smith IR. Histamine release from human right atrium. Br J Pharmacol 1981;74:7.
68. Shore DF, Jones ODH, Rigby ML, Shinebourne EA, Lincoln JCR. Atresia of left atrioventricular connection: Surgical considerations. Br Heart J 1982;47:35.
69. Wheedon D, Shore DF, Lincoln JCR. Continuous monitoring ofpulmonary artery pressure after cardiac surgery in infants and children. J Cardiovasc Surg 1981;22:307.
70. Leijala MA, Lincoln CR, Shinebourne EA, Nellen M. A rare congenital cardiac malformation with situs inversus and discordant atrioventricular and concordant ventriculoarterial connections: Diagnosis and surgical treatment. Am Heart J 1981;101:355.

71. Capuani A, Del Torso S, Lincoln JC. Right lung agenesis: A case report. Giornale Italiano di Cardiologia 1982;12:381.
72. Jones ODH, Shore DF, Rigby ML, Leijala M, Scallan M, Shinebourne EA, Lincoln JCR. The use of tolazoline hydrochloride as a pulmonary vasodilator in potentially fatal pulmonary vasoconstrictive episodes following cardiac surgery in children. Circulation 1981;64:II 134.
73. Shore DF, Ho SY, Anderson RH, de Leval M, Lincoln JCR. Aorto-pulmonary septal defect, co-existing with ventricular septal defect and pulmonary atresia. Ann Thorac Surg 1981;35:132.
74. Rigby ML, Gibson DG, Joseph MC, Lincoln JCR, Shinebourne EA, Shore DF, Anderson RH. The recognition of imperforate atrioventricular valves by two-dimensional echocardiography. Br Heart J 1982;47:329.
75. Shore DF, Capuani A, Lincoln JCR. A typical tamponade after cardiac surgery in infants and children. J Thorac Cardiovasc Surg 1982;83:449.
76. Shore DF, Rigby ML, Lincoln JCR. Severe tricuspid stenosis presenting as tricuspid atresia: Echocardiographic diagnosis and surgical management. Br Heart J 1982;48:404.
77. Al-Faghi Mohammed, Rigby ML, Shinebourne EA, Lincoln JCR. Successful anatomical correction of transposition of the great arteries. Saudi Med J 1982;3:171.
78. Shore DF, Smallhorn J, Stark J, Lincoln JCR, de Leval MR. Left ventricular outflow tract obstruction co-existing with ventricular septal defect. Br Heart J 1982;48:421.
79. Kay PH, Capuani A, Franks R, Lincoln JCR. Experience with modified Blalock Taussig operations using PTFE (Impra) grafts. Br Heart J 1983;49: 359.
80. Firmin RK, Azariades M, Lennox SC, Lincoln JCR, Paneth M. Sleeve lobectomy for bronchial carcinoma. Ann Thor Surg 1983;35:442.
81. Kay P, Mulholland C, Lincoln JCR. A case of congenital double chambered left ventricle treatment by eclusion of the assessory chamber. Br Heart J 1983;49:359.
82. Wells FC, Coghill S, Caplan HL, Lincoln JC. Duration of circulatory arrest does influence the psychological development of children after cardiac operation in early life. J Thorac Cardiovasc Surg 1983;86:823.
83. Pillai R, Shinebourne EA, Anderson RH, Lincoln JCR. Surgical correction in mirror image atrial arrangement or left atrial isomerism with systemic venous return to the left sided atrium. J Thorac Cardiovasc Surg 1983;86: 288.
84. Kay PH, Oldershaw PJ, Lincoln JCR, Lennox SG, Paneth M. The management of prosthetic valve endocarditis. J Cardiovasc Surg 1983;24:127.
85. Lincoln JCR, Lima R, Rigby ML. Anatomical correction of simple trans-

position of the great arteries during neonatal transition. Lancet 1983;2:39 (also Arch Dis Child 1984;59:673).

86. Lane I, Treasure T, Leijala M, Shinebourne E, Lincoln JCR. Diminutive pulmonary artery growth following right ventricular outflow tract enlargement. Int J Cardiol 1983;3:175.
87. Ho SY, Wilcox BR, Anderson RH, Lincoln JCR. Interrupted aortic arch, anatomic features of surgical significance. Thorac Cardiovasc Surg 1983; 31:199.
88. Firmin RK, Lima R, Anderson RH, Ho SY, Lincoln C. Anatomic problems associated with arterial switch procedure for double outlet right ventricle with subpulmonary ventricular septal defect. Thorac Cardiovasc Surg 1983;31:365.
89. Lincoln JCR, Southall D. Cardiac system before and after Mustard' s operation for complete transposition of the great arteries. Pediatr Cardiol 1983;4:165.
90. Pillai R, Ho SY, Anderson RH, Shinebourne EA, Lincoln JCR. Malalignment of the interventricular septum with atrioventricular septal defect: Its implications concerning conducting tissue disposition. Thorac Cardiovasc Surg 1984;32:1.
91. Albuquerque AT, Rigby ML, Anderson RH, Lincoln JCR, Shinebourne EA. The spectrum of atrioventricular discordance: A clinical study. Br Heart J 1984;51:498.
92. Ostman-Smith I, Silverman NH, Oldershaw P, Lincoln JCR, Shinebourne EA. Cor Triatriatum Sinistrum, diagnostic features on cross sectional echocardiography. Br Heart J 1984;51:211.
93. Wilson C, Lincoln C. β-adrenoceptor subtypes in human, rat, guinea pig and rabbit atria. J Cardiovasc Pharmacol 1984;6:1216.
94. Capuani A, Pasque A, Eufrate S, Lincoln JCR. Lo shunt sistemico-polmonare anastomosi di Waterston-Colley versus anastomosi di Blalock-Taussig modificata. Archivio di Chirurgia Toracica e Cardiovascolare. Vol VI- N.I.- Vennaio-Marzo 1984.
95. Baxter P, Rigby ML, Jones ODH, Lincoln JCR, Shinebourne EA. Acute renal failure following cardiopulmonary bypass in children: Results of treatment. Int J Cardiol 1985;7:235.
96. Rossi MB, Ho SY, Anderson RH, Kanter K, Rigby ML, Lincoln JCR. Morphological observations following "anatomical correction" for abnormal ventriculo-arterial connection. Thorac Cardiovasc Surgeon 1985;33: 210.
97. Capuani A, Pasque A, Eufrate S, Pratali S, Lincoln JCR. Importanza delle prostaglandine nel trattamento delle cardiopatie congenite complesse. Arch Chirur Torac Cardiovasc 1985;7:747.

98. Firmin RK, Bouloux P, Allen P, Lima RC, Lincoln JCR. Sympathoadrenal function during cardiac surgery in infants using the technique of surface cooling, limited cardiopulmonary and circulatory arrest. J Thorac Cardiovasc Surg 1985;90:729.
99. Gladstone FJ, Pillai R, Paneth M, Lincoln JCR. Relief of superior vena caval syndrome using autologous femoral vein as a by pass graft. J Thorac Cardiovasc Surg 1985;89:750.
100. Pillai R, Yen Ho S, Anderson RH, Lincoln JCR. Ostium primum AV septal defect: An anatomic and surgical review. Ann Thorac Surg 1986;41: 458.
101. Rossi MB, Ho SY, Anderson RH, Filho RIR, Lincoln JCR. Coronary arteries in complete transposition: The signifcance of the sinus node artery. Ann Thorac Surg 1986;42:573.
102. Kanter K, Rigby ML, Shinebourne EA, Lincoln JCR. Anatomic correction for transposition of the great arteries and double outlet right ventricle. J Thorac Cardiovasc Surg 1985;90:690.
103. Smith LD, Charalmbopoulos C, Rigby ML, Pallisades S, Hunter S, Lincoln C, Shinebourne EA. Discrete sub-aortic stenosis and ventricular septal defect. Arch Dis Child 1985;60:196.
104. Lima RC, Firmin RK, Pillai R, Lennox SC, Cleland WP, Paneth M, Lincoln CR. Surgical management of adults with cyanotic congenital heart disease. Arquivos Brasileiros de Cardiologia 1985;45:175.
105. Kanter K, Anderson RH, Lincoln JCR, Firmin R. Anatomic correction of double outlet right ventricle with subpulmonary ventricular septal defect, the Taussig-Bing anomaly. Ann Thorac Surg 1986;41:287.
106. Crupi G, Pillai R, Parenzan L, Lincoln JCR. Surgical treatment of subpulmonary obstruction in transposition of the great arteries by means of a left ventricular-pulmonary artery arterial conduit. J Thorac Cardiovasc Surg 1985;89:907.
107. Lincoln C, Redington AN, Li K, Mattos S, Shinebourne EAS, Rigby ML. Anatomical correction for complete transposition and double outlet right ventricle: Intermediate account of functional results. Br Heart J 1986; 56:259.
108. Lincoln C, Al-Fagih M, Mercanti C, Joseph M, Miller G, Rigby M, Shinebourne EA. Surgical risk factors in total anomalous pulmonary venous connection. Am J Cardiol 1988;61:608.
109. Richards PG, Marath A, Rice Edwards JM, Lincoln C. Management of difficult intracranial aneurysms by deep hypothermia and elective cardiac arrest using cardiopulmonary bypass. Br J Neurosurgery 1987;1:261.
110. Rossi R, Ekroth R, Lincoln JCR, Jackson A, Thompson R, Scallan M, Tsang V. Detection of cerebral injury after total circulatory arrest and pro-

found hypothermia by estimaton of specifc kinase isoenzyme levels using monoclonal antibody techniques. Am J Cardiol 1986;58:1236.

111. Ekroth R, Rossi RF, Tsang V, Jackson AP, Thompson RJ, Scallan M, Lincoln JCR. Serial measurement of arterial and internal jugular venous creatine kinase isoenzyme BB (CK-BB) after deep hypothermic total circulatory arrest in paediatric cardiac surgery. Thorac Cardiovasc Surgeon 1986;34:223.
112. Lima RC, Firmin RK, Pillai R, Lennox SC, Cleland WP, Paneth M, Lincoln JCR. Surgical management of adults with cyanotic congenital heart disease. Arq Bras Cardiol 1985;45:175.
113. Lincoln C, Rigby M, Cox F, Bossom S. Letter to the Editor. The Times, London. August l0th, 1987.
114. Azariades M, Firmin R, Lincoln JCR, Lennox SC. Cerebral function and analysis during deep hypothermia and total circulatory arrest in infant lambs. Thorac Cardiovasc Surgeon 1988;36:133.
115. Darvell FJ, Rossi IR, Ross MB, Fayers P, Anderson RH, Rigby ML, Shinebourne EA, Lincoln JCR. Intermediate to late term results of Mustard's procedure for complete transposition of the great arteries with an intact ventricular septum. Br Heart J 1988;59:468.
116. Musumeci F, Shumway S, Lincoln JCR, Anderson RH. Surgical treatment for double-outlet right ventricle at the Brompton Hospital, 1973 to 1986. J Thorac Cardiovasc Surg 1988;96:278.
117. Marath A, Richards P, Man W, Taylor KM, Lincoln C, Soni N, Rice-Edwards JM, Bartoli A, Gladstone D. The clinical significance of elevated CSF and plasma histamine in cerebral aneurysm surgery utilizing cardiopulmonary bypass with total circulatory arrest. Agents and Actions 1988;23:343.
118. Marath A, Man W, Taylor KM, Deverall PB, Parsons S, Jones OH, Lincoln C, Kimberly A. Plasma histamine profiles in paediatric cardiopulmonary bypass. Agents and Actions 1988;23:339.
119. Ekroth R, Thompson RJ, Lincoln JCR, Scallan M, Rossi R, Tsang V. Elective deep hypothermia with total circulatory arrest: Changes in plasma creatine kinase BB, blood glucose, clinical variables. J Thorac Cardiovasc Surg 1989;97:30.
120. Kay PH, Brass T, Lincoln JCR. The pathophysiology of atypical tamponade in infants undergoing cardiac surgery. Eur J Cardiothorac Surg 1989;3:255.
121. van der Linden J, Ekroth R, Lincoln JCR, Pugsley W, Scallan M, Tyden H. Is cerebral blood flow/metabolic mismatch during rewarming a risk factor after profound hypothermic procedures in small children? Eur J Cardiothorac Surg 1989;3:209.

122. Rossi R, van der Linden J, Ekroth R, Scallan M, Thompson RJ, Lincoln JCR. No flow or low flow? A study of the ischemic marker creatine kinase BB after deep hypothermic procedures. J Thorac Cardiovasc Surg 1989;98:193.
123. Rossi RF, Ekroth R, Jansson K, Scallan M, Thompson RJ, Lincoln C. Brain type creatine kinase in relation to oxygen desaturation in the blood of children with congenital heart disease. Scand J Thorac Cardiovasc Surg 1990;24:75.
124. Carvalho JS, Busst CM, Redington AN, Lincoln JCR, Rigby ML, Shinebourne EA. Do asymptomatic school children have normal haemodynamics 6–13 years after Mustard's operation? Int J Cardiol 1990;26:259.
125. Boyadjiev K, Ho SY, Anderson RH, Lincoln JCR. The potential for subpulmonary obstruction in complete transposition after the arterial switch procedure. Eur J Cardiothorac Surg 1990;4:214.
126. Azarides M, Firmin R, Lincoln C, Lennox S. The effect of propranolol on the cerebral electrical response to deep hypothermia and total circulatory arrest in lambs. J Thorac Cardiovasc Surg 1990;99:1030.
127. Bowyer J, Busst C, Till J, Lincoln C, Shinebourne E. Exercise ability after Mustard's operation. Arch Dis Child 1990;65:865.
128. Cheung H, Lincoln C, Anderson R, Yen Ho S, Shinebourne E, Pallides S, Rigby M. Options for surgical repair in hearts with univentricular atrioventricular connection and subaortic stenosis. J Thorac Cardiovasc Surg 1990;100:672.
129. Lincoln C. Letter to The Editor. The Times, London. January 10, 1991.
130. Lincoln C, Gibson D, Kay P, Shore D. Delayed sternal closure in neonate. (Letter) J Thorac Cardiovasc Surg 1990;100:928.
131. Carvalho J, Redington A, Oldershaw P, Shinebourne E, Lincoln C, Gibson D. Analysis of left ventricular wall movement before and after reimplantation of anomalous left coronary artery in infancy. Br Heart J 1991;65:218.
132. Lincoln C, Vecht R, Antoniou G, Vironis G. Wellington Hospital-Cyprus High Commission Cardiac Surgical Programme London 1988–1990. Quarterly Publication of The Pancyprian Medical Association.
133. Van der Linden J, Priddy R, Ekroth R, Lincoln C, Pugsley W, Scallan M, Tyden H. Cerebral pertusion and metabolism during profound hypothermia in children. J Thorac Cardiovasc Surg 1991;102:103.
134. Penny D, Lincoln C, Redington A. Abnormal systolic atrioventricular flow related to incoordinate motion of the ventricular wall after Fontan operation. Int J Cardiol 1991;32:112.
135. Burch, Lincoln C, Carter N, Smith A. Acute sternal opening after cardiac surgery in children: Effect on plasma atrial natriuretic peptide. J Cardiovasc Surg 1991;32:246.

136. Bertschmann, Lincoln C. [Arterial switch operation in transposition of great arteries and double-outlet right ventricle. Experience at the Brompton Hospital, London.] [German] Helvetica Chirurgica Acta 1991;57: 545.
137. Penny D, Lincoln C, Shore D, Xiao HB, Rigby M, Redington A. The acute effects of transition to a Fontan circulation. Circulation 1991; 84:513.
138. Penny D, Lincoln C, Xiao H, Rigby M, Redington A. The acute effects of transition to the Fontan circulation on systemic ventricular function. Eur Heart J 1991;12.
139. Lincoln C, Anderson RH. Nomenclatura obscura: Subaortic obstruction in double inlet left ventricle and related lesions. Ann Thorac Surg 1991;52:730.
140. Penny D, Lincoln C, Shore D, Xiao H, Rigby M, Redington A. The early response of the systemic ventricle during transition to the Fontan circulation: An acute hypertrophic cardiomyopathy? Cardiol Young 1992;2:78.
141. Benatar A, Vaughan J, Nicolini U, Corrin B, Lincoln C. Prenatal pericardiocentesis: Its role in the management of intrapericardial teratoma. Obstet Gynaecol 1992;79:856.
142. Ho S, Gerlis LM, Toms J, Lincoln C, Anderson RH. Morphology of the posterior junctional area in atrioventricular septal defects. Ann Thorac Surg 1992;54:264.
143. Van der Linden J, Astudillo R, Ekroth R, Scallan M, Lincoln C. Cerebral lactate release after circulatory arrest but not after low-flow in small children undergoing profound hypothermic procedures. Ann Thorac Surg 1993;56:1485.
144. Millar AB, Armstrong L, Van der Linden J, Moat N, Ekroth R, Westwick J, Lincoln C. Production of cytokines in children undergoing cardiopulmonary bypass: A role for haemofiltration. Ann Thorac Surg 1993;56: 1499.
145. Astudillo R, Van der Linden J, Ekroth R, Wesslen O, Hallhagen S, Scallan M, Shore D, Lincoln C. Absent diastolic cerebral blood flow velocity after circulatory arrest but not after low flow in infants. Ann Thorac Surg 1993;56:515.
146. Peters NS, Severs NJ, Rothery SM, Lincoln C, Yacoub M, Green CR. Spatiotemporal relation between gap junctions and fascia adherens junctions during postnatal development of human ventricular myocardium. Circulation 1994;90:713.
147. Cullen S, Ho SY, Shore D, Lincoln C, Redington A. Congenital stenosis of pulmonary veins: Failure to modify natural history by intra-operative placement of stents. Cardiol Young 1994;4:395–398.

148. Burman JF, Chung HI, Lane DA, Phillippou H, Adami A, Lincoln C. Role of factor XII in thrombin generation and fibrinolysis during cardiopulmonary bypass. Lancet 1994;334:1192.
149. Ekroth R, Van der Linden J, Lincoln C, Scallan M. Cerebral perfusion and metabolism after profound hypothermia: Comparison between procedures involving no flow and low flow. Cardiol Young 1993;3:378.
150. Ross DB, Cheung HC, Lincoln C. Direct relief of subaortic obstruction in patients with univentricular atrioventricular connection and discordant ventriculoarterial connection: Intermediate results. Semin Thorac Cardiovasc Surg 1994;6:33.
151. Chung HI, Burman JF, Balogun BA, Lincoln C, Pepper JR. Elevated fibrinolysis in cardiopulmonary bypass is factor XII dependent. Fibrinolysis 1994;8:84.
152. Shinebourne EA, Jahangiri M, Carvalho JS, Lincoln C. Anatomic correction for post-Mustard pulmonary venous obstruction. Ann Thorac Surg 1994;57:1655.
153. Jahangiri M, Ross DB, Redington A, Lincoln C, Shinebourne EA. Thromboembolism after the Fontan procedure and its modifications. Ann Thorac Surg 1994;58:1409.
154. Saadi EK, Shore D, Lincoln C. Analise dos fatores de risco na correcao cirurgica do defeito septal atrioventricular de forma total. Rev Bras Circ Cardiovasc 1993;8:136.
155. Vogel M, Siew YH, Lincoln C, Yacoub MH, Anderson RH. Three-dimensional echocardiography can simulate intraoperative visualization of congenitally malformed hearts. Ann Thorac Surg 1995;60:1282.
156. Scallan M, Lincoln C. Invited commentary on: Kern FH, Ungerleider RM, Scott RS, et al. Comparing two strategies of cardiopulmonary bypass cooling on jugular venous oxygen saturation in neonates and infants. Ann Thorac Surg 1995;60.
157. Shekerdemian LS, Shore DF, Lincoln C, Bush A, Redington AN. Negative pressure ventilation improves the cardiac output after right heart surgery. Circulation 1996;94:II 49.
158. Moraes F, Lincoln C. Anomalous origin of the left coronary artery: Evolution of surgical treatment. Eur J Cardiothorac Surg 1996;10:603.
159. White P, Chaturvedi R, Shore D, Lincoln C, Szwarc RS, Bishop AJ, Oldershaw PJ, Redington A. Left ventricular parallel conductance during the cardiac cycle in children with congenital heart disease. Am J Physiol 1997;273:H 295.
160. Jahangiri M, Shore D, Kakkar V, Shinebourne E, Lincoln C. Coagulation factor abnormalities following the Fontan procedure and its modifications. J Thorac Cardiovasc Surg 1997;113:989.

161. Nicholson A, Rigby M, Lincoln C, Miller S, Fisher C. Synovial sarcoma of the heart in a 13 year old boy. Histopathology 1997;30:349.
162. Norgard G, Gatzoulis MA, Morales F, Lincoln C, Shore DF, Shinebourne EA, Redington AN. The relationship between type of repair and right ventricular diastolic physiology in post-operative tetralogy of Fallot: Implications for long term outcome. Circulation 1996;94:3276.
163. Lincoln C. Invited comment—Rodriguez RA, Austin EH, Audenaert SM. Postbypass effects of delayed rewarming on cerebral blood flow velocities in infants after total circulatory arrest. J Thorac Cardiovasc Surg 1995;110:1686.
164. Taggart DP, Hadjinikolaou L, Hooper J, Lincoln C, Yacoub M. Troponin-T in cardiac surgery [letter; comment]. Ann Thorac Surg 1996;61:1040.
165. Taggart DP, Hadjinikolaou L, Wong K, Yap J, Hooper J, Kemp M, Hue D, Yacoub M, Lincoln C. Vulnerability of paediatric myocardium to cardiac surgery. Heart 1996;76:214.
166. Taggart DP, Hadjinikolaou L, Hooper J, Albert J, Kemp M, Hue D, Yacoub M, Lincoln C. Effects of age and ischaemic times on biochemical evidence of myocardial injury after paediatric cardiac operations. J Thorac Cardiovasc Surg 1997;113:728.
167. Al-Zaghal AN, Li J, Anderson RH, Lincoln C, Shore DS, Rigby ML. Anatomic criteria for the diagnosis of sinus venosus defects. Heart 1997; 78:298.
168. Roberts CS, Peters P, Lincoln C. Right heart bypass using an extracardiac conduit for functionally single ventricle with anomalous pulmonary venous connection to the right atrium. J Thorac Cardiovasc Surg 1997; 114:297.
169. Chaturvedi RR, White P, Lincoln C, Redington AN, Shore D. Left ventricular dysfunction after repair of simple congenital heart defects in infants and children: Quantitation using a conductance catheter immediately after bypass. J Thorac Cardiovasc Surg 1998;115:77.
170. Shekerdemian LS, Bush A, Shore D, Lincoln C, Redington AN. Cardiopulmonary interactions after Fontan operations: Augmentation of cardiac output using negative pressure ventilation. Circulation 1997;96: 3934.
171. Shekerdemian LS, Bush A, Lincoln C, Shore D, Petros AJ, Redington AN. Cardiopulmonary interactions in healthy children and children after simple cardiac surgery: The effects of positive and negative pressure ventilation. Heart 1997;78:587.
172. Mayet J, Kanagaratnam P, Lincoln C, Oldershaw P. Hypereosinophilic syndrome: Endomyocardial fibrosis [letter; comment]. Heart 1997; 77:391.
173. Lincoln C. Right heart bypass with an extracardiac conduit: A cautionary tale [letter]. J Thorac Cardiovasc Surg 1998;115:964.

Book Chapters

1. Lincoln JCR. Aspects of the surgery of non-malignant pulmonary disease. In: Respiratory Disease. Lane, ed. London: William Heinemann Medical Books, 1976.
2. Jamieson SW, Lincoln C. Some effects of sulphinpyrazone cardiac bypass surgery. In: Thrombo-Embolism: A New Approach to Therapy. Mitchel, ed. London: Academic Press, 1977.
3. Lincoln C. Surgery of corrected transposition in situs inversus. In: Paediatric Cardiology. Anderson, ed. Edinburgh: Churchill Livingstone, 1978.
4. Lincoln JCR. Transatrial versus transventricular closure of isolate ventricular septal defect. In: Paediatric Cardiology. Anderson, ed. Edinburgh: Churchill Livingstone, 1978.
5. Lincoln C. Complete intra-cardiac repair of Fallot's tetralogy. In: Operative Surgery. Jackson, ed. London: Butterworths, 1978.
6. Lincoln, C, Capuani A, Shinebourne EA. Primary surgical treatment of ventricular septal defect under three months and between 3–6 months of life. Parenzan, ed. Bologna: Patron Editore, 1980.
7. Lincoln C. The surgical principles and treatments of neonatal infants with congenital heart disease. In: Scientific Foundations of Cardiology. Sleight, ed. London: William Heinemann Medical Books, 1983.
8. Franks R, Lincoln C. Management of double outlet right ventricle. In: Paediatric Cardiology. Anderson, ed. Edinburgh: Churchill Livingstone, 1983.
9. Lincoln C, Crupi G. Congenital heart disease. In: Surgical Management. Taylor, ed. London: William Heinemann Medical Books, 1984.
10. Lincoln C. Tamponamento Cardiaco Tratamento Intensivo Pos-Operatorio. Lucchese, ed. Sao Paulo: Fundo Editorial Byk-Proåenx, 1985.
11. Lincoln C. Tetralogy of Fallot: Surgical treatment. In: Operative Surgery. Rob, ed. London: Butterworths, 1986.
12. Lincoln JCR, Scallan M. Congenital heart disease. In: Surgery for Anaesthetists. Zorab, ed. Oxford: Blackwell Scientific Publications, 1988.
13. Lincoln C. Anomalous pulmonary venous connection. In: Current Therapy in Cardiothoracic Surgery. Grillo, ed. Toronto: B.C. Decker, Inc., 1989.
14. Lincoln C. Total anomalous pulmonary venous connection. Perspectives in Pediatric Cardiology, Vol. 2, Pediatric Cardiac Surgery, Part 2. Crupi G, ed. New York: Futura Publishing Company, 1989.

Appendix II

Christopher Lincoln FRCS Fellows in Paediatric Cardiac Surgery: Royal Brompton Hospital

1977	C. Krayenbuhl	Switzerland
1978	G. Crupi	Italy
1979	M. Leijala	Finland
1980	A. Capuani	Italy
1981	M. Al-Fagigh	Saudi Arabia
1982	R. Lima	Brazil
1983	C. Mercanti	Italy
1983	R. Ekroth	Sweden
1984	K. Kantor	U.S.A.
1985	A. Rossi	Brazil
1986	S. Shumway	U.S.A
1986	F. Musumecci	Italy
1987	B. Urso	Italy
1988	H. Cheung	Hong Kong
1989	J. Dien	U.S.A.
1989	W. Bertschmann	Switzerland
1990	M. Teodori	U.S.A.
1991	E. Saadi	Brazil
1991	R. Lowell	U.S.A.
1991	R. Scarbieri	Brazil
1991	O. Wesslen	Sweden
1992	D. Ross	Canada
1993	P. Medeiros	Brazil
1993	P. Lertpradit	Thailand
1994	L. Hadjinikolaou	Greece
1994	F. Moraes	Brazil
1996	C. Roberts	U.S.A.

Appendix III

Right Heart Bypass with an Extracardiac Conduit for Functionally Single Ventricle with Anomalous Pulmonary Venous Connection to the Right Atrium

Charles S. Roberts, MD, Paul Peters, FRCS, and Christopher Lincoln, FRCS, *London, United Kingdom*

Several methods for bypassing the right side of the heart have been reported in the past 40 years. Our usual technique is total cavopulmonary connection as described by de Leval and associates[1] in 1988. Herin we present the case history of a child with a functionally single ventricle and totally anomalous pulmonary venous drainage to the right atrium, which necessitated an unusual technique.

Clinical summary. A 2-year-old child was referred to the Royal Brompton Hospital with cyanotic complex congenital heart disease. She had been cyanotic from birth, had become increasingly breathless, and had recurrent chest infections. She had clubbing of the fingers and toes and a loud precordial systolic murmur. Echocardiography and cardiac catheterization revealed bilateral superior venae cavae (SVCs) and a single right-sided inferior vena cava (IVC), isomerism of the right atrial appendages with a large atrial septal defect, a univentricular atrioventricular connection via a common atrioventricular valve to a dominant right ventricle, a hypoplastic left ventricle, double-outlet right ventricle with pulmonary stenosis, and totally anomalous pulmonary venous connection

From the Royal Brompton Hospital, Sydney Street, London, United Kingdom.
Received for publication Jan. 22, 1997; accepted for publication Feb. 10, 1997.
Address for reprints: Christopher Lincoln, FRCS, Royal Brompton Hospital, Sydney Street, London SW3 6NP, United Kingdom.
J Thorac Cardiovasc Surg 1997;114:297–8

0022-5223/97 $5.00 + 0 **12/54/81122**

to the right atrium, near the orifice of the SVC. She did not have subaortic stenosis, and the mean pulmonary arterial pressure was 11 mm Hg.

A conventional total cavopulmonary connection was attempted. Bilateral bidirectional Glenn shunts were constructed. A lateral intraatrial baffle was placed to direct IVC blood to the pulmonary arteries, attempting to avoid the pulmonary venous connection in the right atrium. Nevertheless, when cardiopulmonary bypass was being discontinued, it became evident that pulmonary venous return was obstructed. The baffle was therefore taken down. Postoperatively, right upper lobe consolidation occurred because of apparent obstruction of the pulmonary vein to the lobe. Otherwise, recovery was uneventful and the child was discharged with an arterial oxygen saturation of 80%.

At the age 3 years 10 months, the child underwent a second echocardiogram and cardiac catheterization. The bilateral bidirectional Glenn shunts were patent, mean pulmonary arterial pressure was 9 mm Hg, and ventricular function was good. Arterial oxygen saturation was 86%. A second operation was undertaken. With the use of a predominantly extracardiac conduit (19 mm polytetrafluoroethylene tube graft), IVC blood was directed to the pulmonary arteries (Fig. 1). The proximal end of the tube graft was sewn to the IVC orifice in the right atrium. A fenestration 4 mm in diameter was made in the tube graft within the right atrium. The tube graft was then brought out through the right lateral wall of the right atrium and its distal end was sewn to the central portion of the right pulmonary artery (medial to the right bidirectional Glenn anastomosis). By creating a primarily extracardiac pathway for IVC flow to the pulmonary arteries, we avoided the anomalous pulmonary venous connection in the upper right atrium. A patch was used to enlarge the right posterolateral aspect of the confluence of the pulmonary veins.

Postoperative recovery was uneventful except for development of bilateral pleural effusions, which necessitated drainage. Echocardiography showed no obstruction to systemic or pulmonary venous pathways and good ventricular function. Arterial oxygen saturations were above 90% and the child was discharged to her home after 21 hospital days.

Discussion. Total cavopulmonary connection was our operative goal in this child with a functionally single ventricle. Our usual technique was not possible, however, because of the pulmonary venous connection to the right atrium near the orifice of the SVC. The predominantly extracardiac conduit avoided the potential obstruction of pulmonary venous return.

In 1990 Marcelletti and associates[2] described four patients who

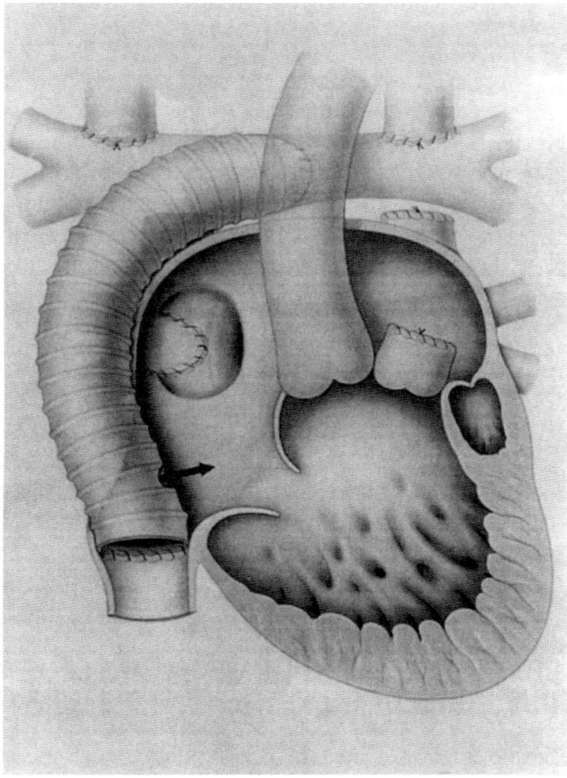

Fig. 1. Total cavopulmonary connection using a predominantly extracardiac conduit in a child with a functionally single ventricle and anomalous pulmonary venous connection to the right atrium. A 4 mm fenestration was made in the intraatrial portion of the conduit.

were treated by placing an extracardiac conduit from the IVC to the pulmonary arteries.[2] One had similar but not identical anatomy to our patient. A further 28 cases were reported in 1992, none of which involved anomalous pulmonary venous connection to the right atrium.[3] The technique of creating a fenestration in the tube graft in its intraatrial portion was recommended to us by de Leval in a personal communcation. A different technique of fenestration has been described by Black and associates,[4] who interposed a small tube graft between the extracardiac conduit and the right atrium.

REFERENCES

1. de Leval MR, Kilner P, Gewillig M, Bull C. Total cavopulmonary connection: a logical alternative to atriopulmonary connection for complex Fontan operations—experimental studies and early clinical experience. J Thorac Cardiovasc Surg 1988;96;682–95.
2. Marcelletti C, Corno A, Giannico S, Marino B. Inferior vena cava- pulmonary artery extracardiac conduit: a new form of right heart bypass. J Thorac Cardiovasc Surg 1990;100:228–32.
3. Giannico S, Corno A, Marino B, Cicini MP, Cagliardi MG, Amodeo A, et a]. Total extracardiac right heart bypass. Circulation 1992;86(Supp 1):II110–7.
4. Black MD, van Son JAM, Haas GS. Extracardiac Fontan operation with adjustable communication. Ann Thorac Surg 1995;60:716–8.

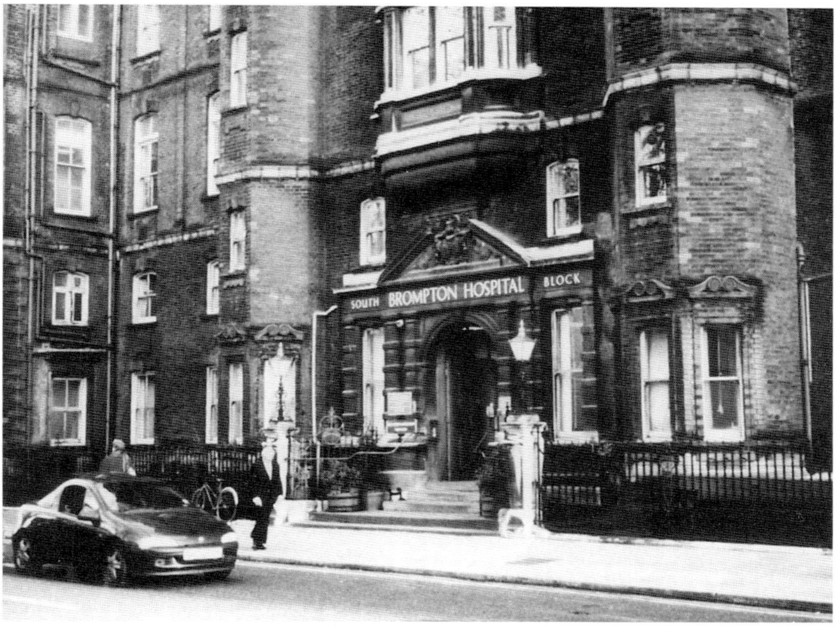

The South Block building of the old Brompton Hospital on Fulham Road. Lincoln's Monday afternoon clinic was held on the first floor. The new Royal Brompton Hospital opened on Sydney Street in 1990.

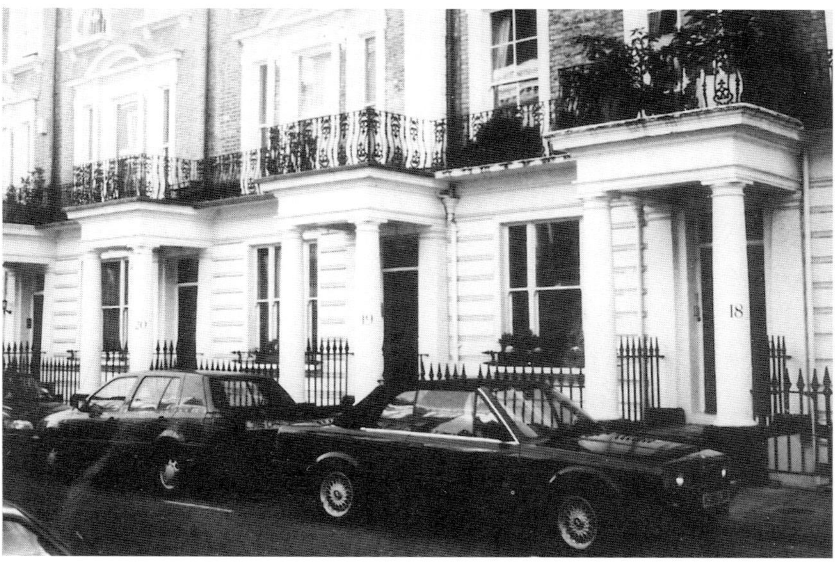

My home for about five months was 19 Neville Street, one block from the Hospital. I rented the front room at street level. Haznat Khan, who achieved notoriety during the year because he dated Lady Diana, lived next door at 20 Neville Street.

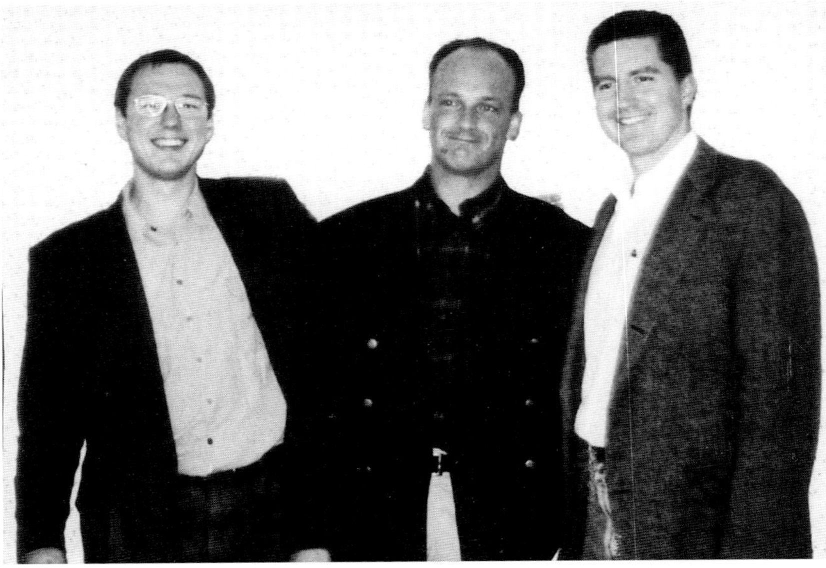

The East German on the left is Stefan Anker, a physician from East Berlin. He lived in the basement flat and worked long hours on his research in heart failure. The West German in the middle is Christoph Stamm who was a surgical trainee from Göttingen University working in the cardiac morphology unit of Professor Robert Anderson. The two Germans were as different as night and day.

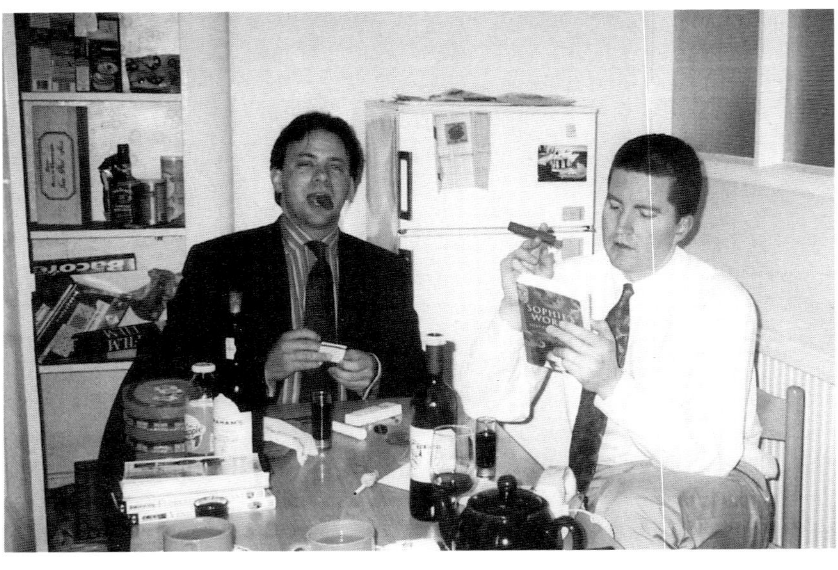

Francis Ferdinand and I were enjoying Cohiba cigars and Graham's port. The bold-striped English shirt worn by Ferdinand was purchased on our foray to Jermyn Street with Lincoln. I did not immediately abandon Brooks Brothers.

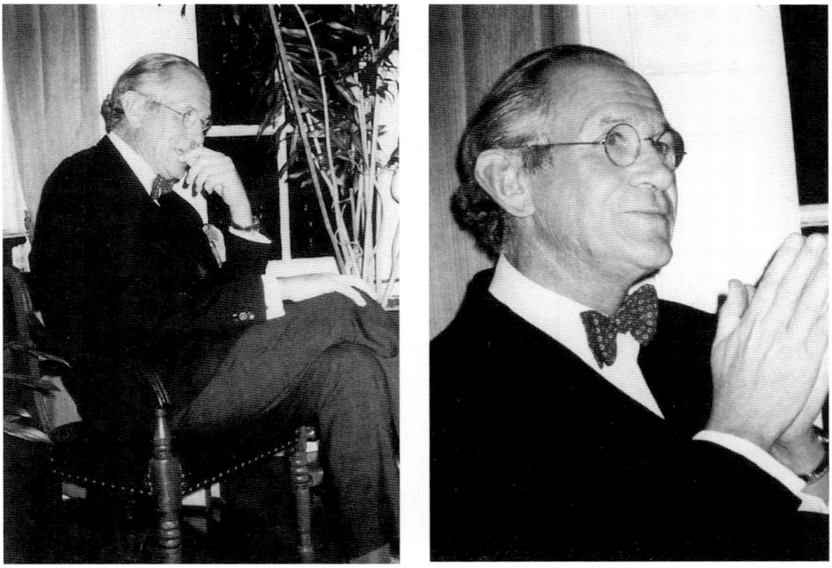

Mr. Christopher Lincoln in his front parlor at Pembroke Square.

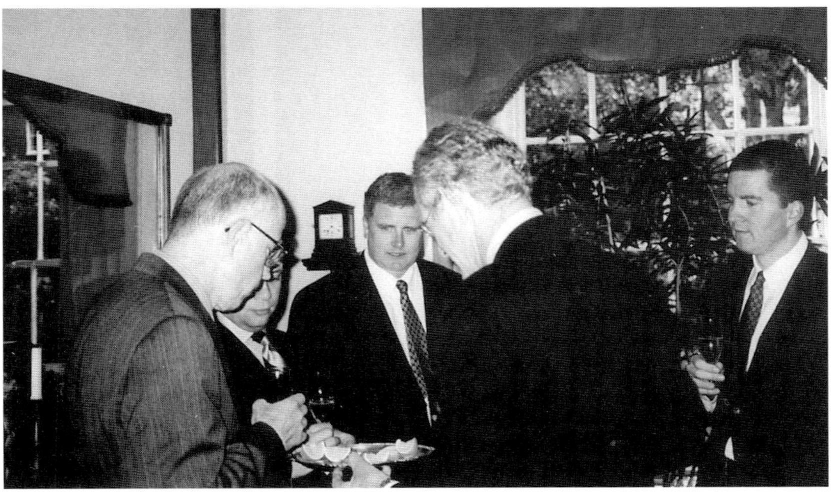

William Roberts, Francis Ferdinand, Clifford Roberts, Christopher Lincoln, and the author sampling the salmon rolls with lemon at Lincoln's home.

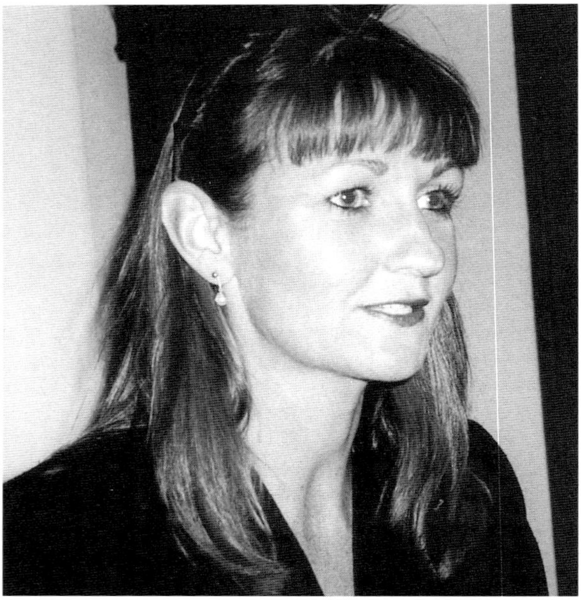

Karen Jurgens, the South African surgical assistant on our team, at Lincoln's home in the spring.

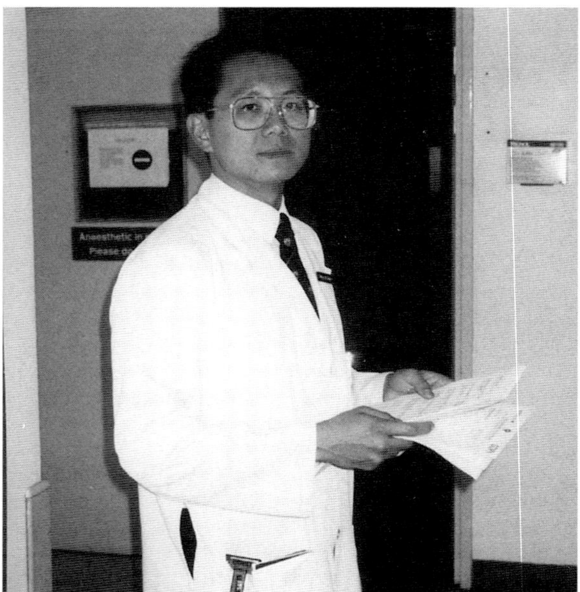

Tony Desouza on his way to see patients.

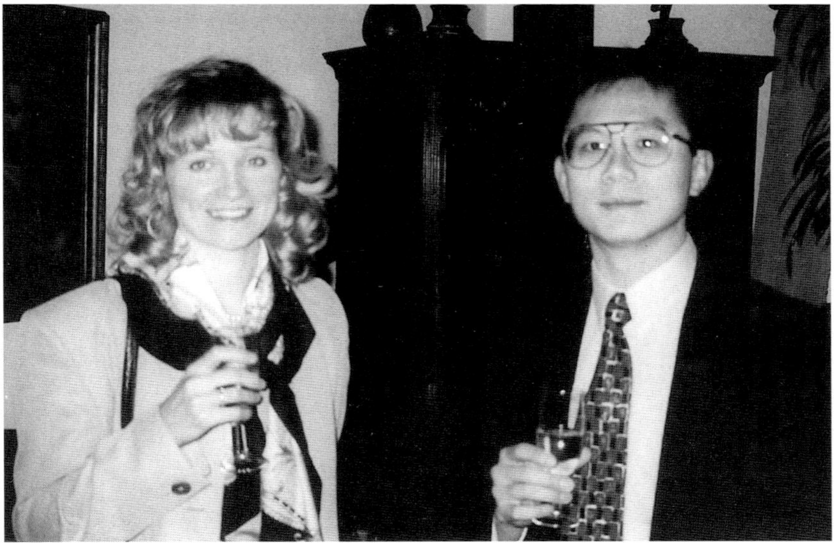

Sarah and Tony Desouza drinking champagne at Lincoln's home. My six months with Tony on Lincoln's team were the most enjoyable months in my ten years of training. He was a superb surgeon.

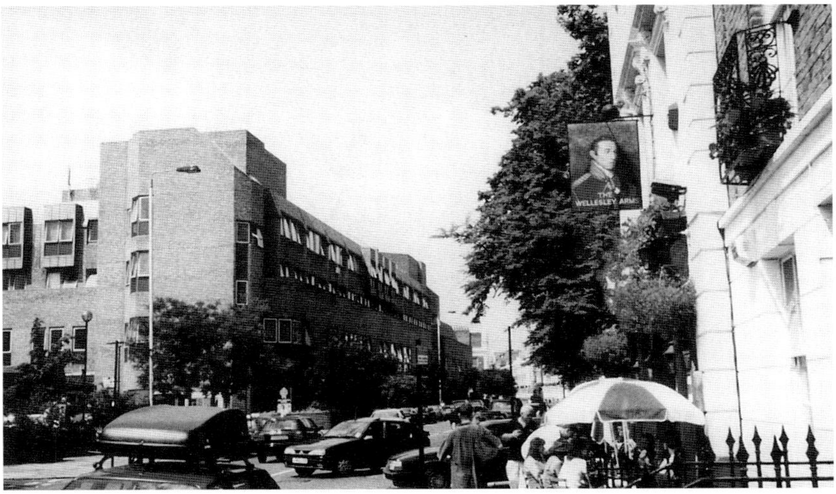

The Wellesley Arms Pub was strategically positioned directly across the street from the Royal Brompton Hospital. Nurses, secretaries, surgical assistants, and doctors often met there after work.

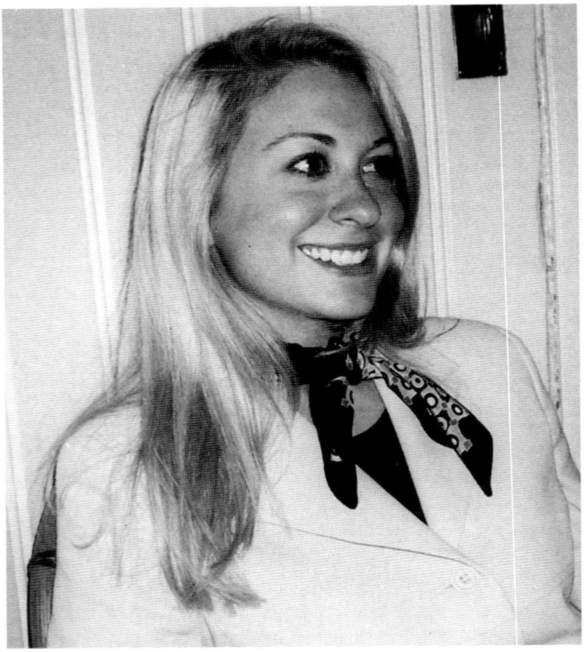

Mary Lydia Warren, my fiancée, at Hilliards Restaurant on Old Brompton Road.

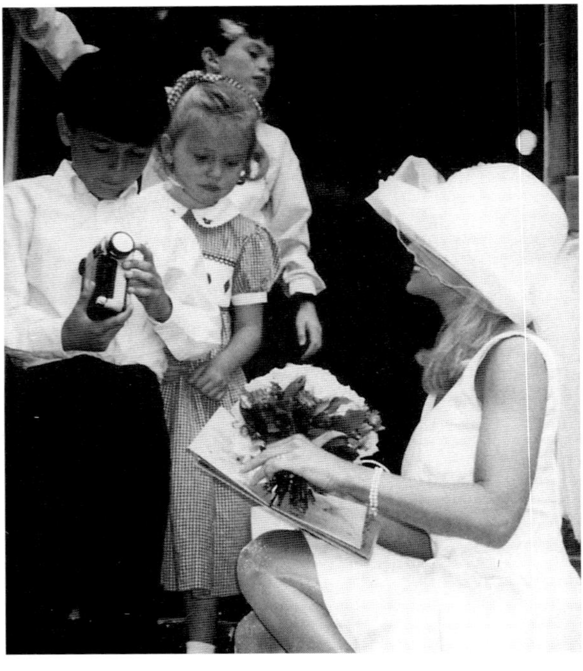

Lydia Warren Roberts on our wedding day with the three Spencer children she sometimes looked after during her four months in London.

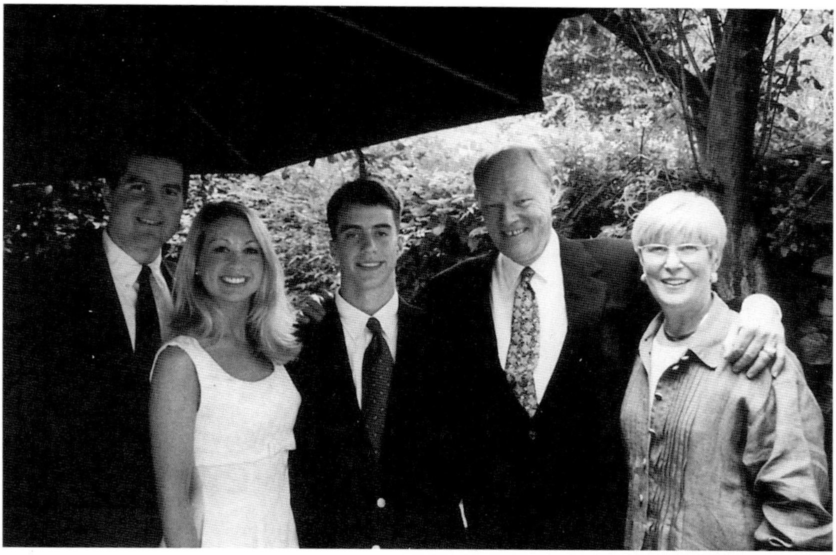

The author, Lydia, David Warren, and our dear friends Cyrus and Judy Wilson. I was a frequent visitor to their home on Park Walk in Chelsea. In fact, I lived there the month of December, when they returned briefly to the States.

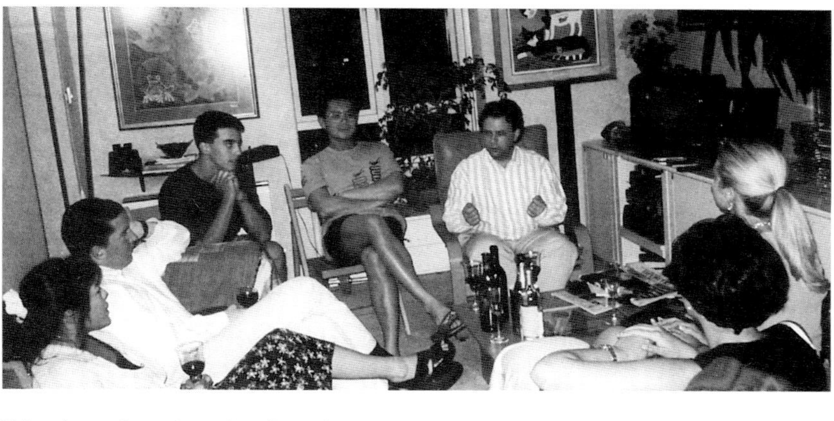

Friends gathered at the flat of Tony and Sarah Desouza in Fulham. Francis Ferdinand is holding court.

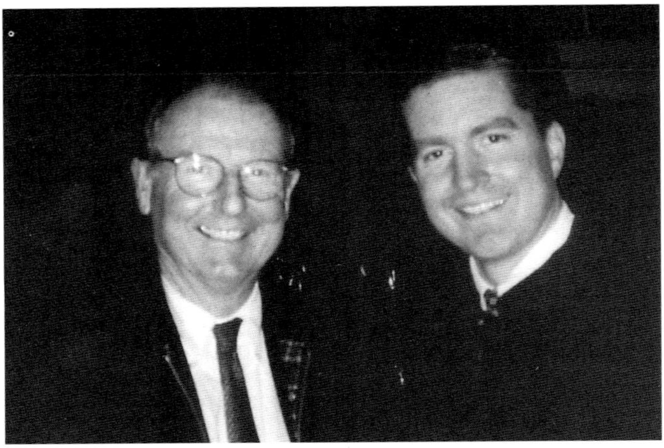

Dr. Benson R. Wilcox, my chief at The University of North Carolina in Chapel Hill, and I standing in front of a plaque which read "This is the home and museum of Dr. William Hunter, Anatomist, 1718–1783."

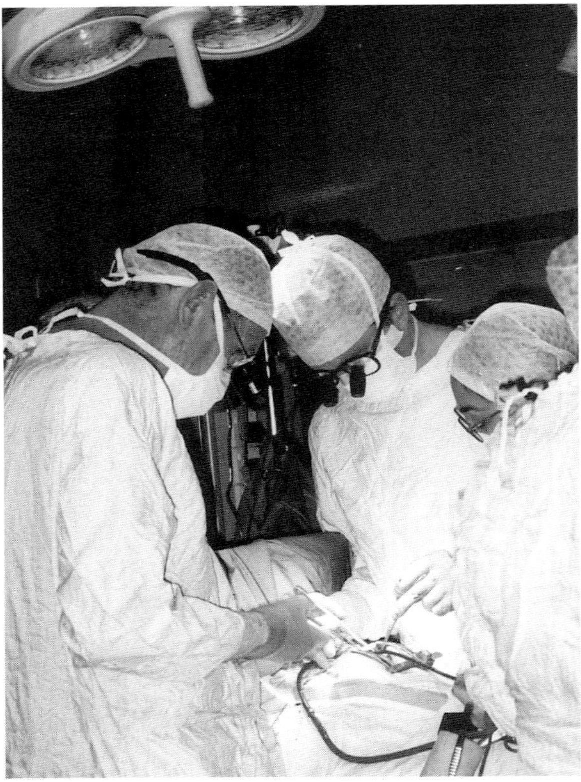

Lincoln (left) and the author operating on a child together.